Practical
Government
Budgeting

SUNY Series in Public Administration
Peter W. Colby, Editor

Practical Government Budgeting

A Workbook for Public Managers

Susan L. Riley and Peter W. Colby

STATE UNIVERSITY OF NEW YORK PRESS

Published by
State University of New York Press, Albany

For information address State University of New York Press,
 194 Washington Avenue, Suite 305, Albany, NY 12210-2384

Library of Congress Cataloging-in-Publication Data

Riley, Susan L., 1952-
    Practical government budgeting : a workbook for public managers /
Susan L. Riley and Peter W. Colby.
        p. cm. — (SUNY series in public administration)
    Includes bibliographical references.
    ISBN 0-7914-0391-2 (alk. paper). — ISBN 0-7914-0392-0 (alk. paper
    : pbk.)
    1. Local budgets—United States. 2. Program budgeting—United
States. I. Colby, Peter W. II. Title. III. Series.
HJ9147.R55 1991
352. 1′ 22042′ 0973—dc20   89-26374
                                                              CIP

10 9 8 7 6 5 4 3 2 1

CONTENTS _____

EXHIBITS   ——————————————————————

PREFACE

There are many fine textbooks available for Public Administration courses in the field of Public Budgeting. These books provide an excellent picture of budget theory and the intricacies of financial management, especially as they apply to the federal government.

However, we believe that there is a definite lack of teaching materials for the Public Budgeting courses which are directed towards public managers rather than scholars or budget officials. In particular, there is a need for materials designed for the present and future state and (especially) local government officials and staff who comprise the vast majority of students in many Master of Public Administration (MPA) programs.

The co-authors of this volume are a former practitioner who is now a college instructor and an academic who has considerable experience in local government as a trainer, consultant, and former elected official. Together, we team-teach a required MPA-level Public Budgeting course.

Our experiences in government and the classroom have convinced us that many MPA students and programs would benefit from a supplementary workbook emphasizing practical knowledge for state and local government managers. Such a book should take public administration students step by step through the budget techniques they will need to function successfully in line or staff positions throughout state and local government. Few students in MPA programs are or will become either professors or budget officials, but most will have to deal with preparing budget recommendations, requesting new personnel or equipment, estimating revenues collected by their agency, and tracking spending versus budget allocations through the fiscal year.

A nationwide survey of public budgeting practitioners conducted during 1985 and 1986 (source: Daniel E. O'Toole and James Marshall, "Budgeting Practices in Local Government: the State of the Art," *Government Finance Review*, October 1987, pp. 11-15) indicated that:

- the organization of the budget function at the local level typically involves the use of a budget office

- staff judgement founded on expertise and experience plus trend projections based on historical data are the most often used techniques for preparing revenue and expenditure estimates

- the line-item budget format is by far the most commonly used.

It is our intention in this workbook to address this existing state of the art in subnational budgeting. While we recognize the importance of acquainting MPA students with advanced technique and sophisticated theory, the purpose here is to help students acquire the knowledge, skills, and abilities to master local government budgeting as it is actually practiced.

Each chapter of this book is divided into three distinct sections:

 The first section of each chapter is an introduction to the subject matter, stressing how the chapter should be useful to public managers and outlining the specific objectives to be achieved through working with the chapter. The first section also explains how that chapter relates to the entire budget process.

The next section of each chapter requires the active participation of readers in order to learn the techniques of the budget process. Numerous exhibits, terms and concepts, and step-by-step demonstrations are designed to assist readers in becoming familiar with and being able to utilize budget techniques which are helpful, practical, and actually used in most local governments.

 The third and final section of each chapter is devoted to one or more exercises to enable readers to test whether they have acquired the knowledge, skills, or abilities that the chapter includes. These exercises range from mathematical problems to role-plays to demonstrating good "budget judgement" in various political situations. These exercises will help readers master chapter contents.

Students of public budgeting should find this book relevant, practical, and useful. A combination of this workbook with any of the major budgeting texts on the market will provide the foundation for a much stronger Public Budgeting course for students pursuing careers in government administration outside Washington, D.C.

ACKNOWLEDGMENTS _____

We would like to acknowledge the work of Jan C. McLarty who drew the cartoons appearing in this volume and, also, the cooperation of the Council of State Governments which granted permission to use earlier versions of these cartoons which appeared in S. Kenneth Howard, *Changing State Budgeting* (Lexington, Kentucky: Council of State Governments, 1973). Also, a version of Exhibit 8-2 in this volume appeared in *A Capital Improvement Programming Handbook* (Chicago, Illinois: Municipal Finance Officers Association, 1979), p. viii.

Many of the exhibits in this volume are based upon examples found in various noncopyrighted public documents issued by state and local governments. Most have been modified for educational purposes. Among the many jurisdictions whose documents we have used, we particularly would like to acknowledge the use of materials from the State of Florida; Orange County, Florida; and Volusia County, Florida.

Chapter 1

HOW TO READ A GOVERNMENT BUDGET _____

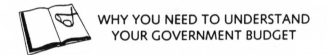

WHY YOU NEED TO UNDERSTAND
YOUR GOVERNMENT BUDGET

HOW THIS CHAPTER WILL BE USEFUL

A local government's budget is the most effective tool available to communicate its fiscal and management policies. The budget document is the governmental entity's detailed financial plan of estimated revenues and expenditures for a specific period of time, normally for 12 months.

In order to understand a budget, the reader needs to know what type of data is contained in the budget document, as well as why it is in the document. Budget documents vary in size, format, and thickness depending on the preference of the governing body or elected officials. However, a local government budget is usually a very thick document that contains reams of valuable information about the government's operations. Nonethless, if one does not understand how to use the data, the document is of little value to the reader or to those who compiled the document.

In an effort to enable the reader to more easily understand the budget document and its composition, we will describe the types of governmental budgets and funds used in public sector accounting, as well as the basic elements of a budget document. Before beginning, however, the reader should become familiar with budget terms and concepts. Some of the most relevant definitions for this chapter are found in Exhibit 1-1.

OBJECTIVES

The main objectives of this chapter are to enable you to:

1. Identify the three types of budgets utilized by local governments in preparing their annual budget.

| Exhibit 1-1 | **Budget Document Terms and Concepts** |

o **Assessed valuation** is the value placed on property for the purpose of distributing the tax burden.

o **Budget** is a financial plan, including estimated revenues and expenditures, for a specific period of time. The **adopted budget** is approved by the legislature prior to the start of the fiscal year; a **revised budget** may be approved during the fiscal year if necessary.

o **Budget document** is the instrument used to present a governmental jurisdictions' comprehensive financial plan.

o **Expenditure** is the disbursement of money to cover the expenses of a governmental agency's operations.

o **Fiscal year** is the 12-month period in which a governmental agency operates. For example, the fiscal year (FY) from October 1, 1988 through September 30, 1989 would be considered either FY 88-89 or simply, FY 89.

    o **Budget year:** fiscal year for which the budget is being considered; fiscal year following the current year
    o **Current year:** fiscal year in progress.
    o **Prior year:** fiscal year preceding the current year.

In most budget documents, **prior year** figures are **actual** spending or revenues, **current year** numbers are **estimates** based on the year-to-date, and **budget year** data reflect **plans** for the future.

o **Fund** is an accounting device established to control the receipt and disbursement of income.

 Millage rate is the tax rate expressed in mills per dollar; i.e., 1 mill equals $1 per $1000 of assessed valuation.

o **Object codes** are specific numerical classifications for which money is allocated for disbursements (expenditures).

o **Revenue** is the money received by a governmental agency to operate. Also referred to as collections or receipts.

o **Revenue sources** are specific areas from which revenue is derived, i.e. ad valorem taxes, utility use fees, beach tolls, etc.

2. Identify the three categories of funds used by governmental jurisdictions in accounting for revenues and expenditures.

3. Describe the four basic elements of a budget document.

READING AND
UNDERSTANDING THE BUDGET

Three Types of Budgets

In preparing budgets, local governments normally utilize one of the following types: line-item, program, or performance. A budget may be a combination of more than one budget type. Normally,

Exhibit 1-2   Three Types of Budgets

Budget Type	Characteristics	Question	Orientation / Criterion
Line item	Expenditures and revenues related to commodities	What is to be bought?	Control / Economy
Program	Expenditures and revenues related to public goals	What is to be achieved?	Planning / Effectiveness
Performance	Expenditures and revenues related to workloads	What is to be done?	Management / Efficiency

government budgets are planned and approved on a detailed line-item basis. However, monies may be controlled and managed on a broader, less detailed level. Each type, however, differs in the way in which monies are allocated for expenditures and in the orientation of the budget: control, management, or planning (see Exhibit 1-2).[1] *a VAWA Grant*

A **line-item budget** is one in which monies are allocated to specific items or objects of cost. Cost categories include personal services, operating expenses, and capital outlay. These cost categories are often further detailed in terms of object codes. For example, personal services can be broken down into salaries, retirement, and health insurance costs, while operating expenses would include such items as office supplies, printing, and utility costs. The cost category capital outlay includes office equipment, furniture, and vehicles.

The main orientation of a line-item budget is that of expenditure control and accountability. This type of budget is easy to prepare and shows how much money is appropriated to a specific cost category. However, it does not provide any information regarding the activities or functions of a program, department, or organization. An example of a line-item budget follows:

Line Item Budget
FY 1988 - 89 Expenditures

ITEM	
Personal Services	
Salaries	$50,000
Retirement	5,000
Insurance	2,500
	$57,500

ITEM	
Operating Expenses	
Office supplies	$ 1,000
Printing	500
	$ 1,500
Capital Outlay	
Desk, chairs	$ 650
TOTAL	$59,650

A **program budget** allocates money to major program areas or activities rather than to specific line items. Program areas often utilized by governmental entities might include public safety, public works, human services, leisure services, and general government. Program areas are related to an organization's goals and often cross organizational lines. For example, public safety is considered a single public concern, however, it includes two distinct and separate program activities—fire and police protection. The main orientation of this budget type is that of planning a budget in a manner that allows for improved decision making regarding the organization's goals. A program budget follows the form detailed here:

Program Budget
FY 1988 - 89 Expenditures

Public Safety	
Fire Protection	$1,000,000
Police Protection	1,800,000
	$2,800,000
Leisure Services	
Parks and Recreation	$ 500,000
Library Services	750,000
	$1,250,000
TOTAL	$4,050,000

A **performance budget** allocates money to various programs within an organization but also details the service level on which the budget is predicated. Service level is identified by the use of performance measures/statistics. The main budget orientation of the performance budget is that of improving internal mangement of the program, as well as seeking to control the costs of the program. A performance budget is illustrated as follows:

ROAD MAINTENANCE
PERFORMANCE MEASURES/STATISTICS

Paving Roads
> Number of miles to pave: 10 miles
> Cost per mile to pave: $300,000 per mile
> Total Annual Cost: $3,000,000

Resurfacing Roads
> Number of miles to resurface: 5 miles
> Cost per mile to resurface: $150,000
> Total Annual Cost: $ 750,000

TOTAL $3,750,000

Three Types of Funds

Local governments are required to account for the receipt and expenditure of all monies received on behalf of the jurisdiction. Such financial records are generally divided into several funds.[2] As defined by the Generally Accepted Accounting Principles (GAAP), a fund is a set of interrelated accounts which record assets (revenues) and liabilities (expenditures/obligations) related to a specific purpose. There are three basic types of funds utilized by governmental agencies: governmental, proprietary, and fiduciary.

Governmental Funds are the first category, usually including the bulk of the budget. These funds account for all records of operations not normally found in business:

- The **General Fund** is comprised of such general revenue sources as taxes, fines, licenses, and fees. One General Fund exists per government and is usually the largest fund utilized.

- **Special Revenue Funds** contain resources that are legally restricted for specific purposes.

    Examples: Transportation Trust Fund
    Library Fund
    State and Federal Grant Funds

- **Debt Service Funds** account for the monies used to repay long-term, generally obligated debt.

    Examples: Library Debt Service
    General Obligation Bonds

- **Capital Project Funds** contain money restricted for construction and acquisition of major capital facilities.

> Examples: Courthouse Complex Renovation
> Library Construction

- **Special Assessment Funds** contain monies received from special charges levied on property owners who benefit from a particular capital improvement or service.

> Examples: Street Lighting Districts
> Road Improvement Assessment Projects

Exhibit 1-3   Length May Vary

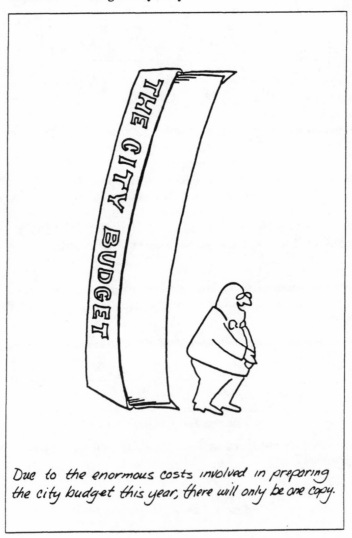

Due to the enormous costs involved in preparing the city budget this year, there will only be one copy.

Proprietary Funds are the second major fund type. These funds account for records of operations similar to those found in a business, such as:

- **Enterprise Funds** contain financial records of self-supporting operations.

  Examples: Water and Sewer Fund
  Solid Waste Fund
  Regional Airport Fund

- **Internal Service Funds** account for the financing of goods or services provided by one department or agency to other departments or governmental agencies on a cost-reimbursement basis.

  Examples: Data Processing
  Building Maintenance
  Reproduction Services

Exhibit 1-4   A Sample Budget Message

Ocean County

July 20, 1989

Board of County Commissioners
Ocean County

Dear Commissioners:

The FY88 County budget of $521 million anticipates a very ambitious work plan by all branches of the government. I'm sure you will agree that we have focused our attention and County resources on the areas of greatest concern to our citizens. As a result, during the next fiscal year we will make substantial progress toward attainment of the goals I've articulated: our customer service will be improved; capital projects will be completed more rapidly; we will be more cost effective; and our community's attractiveness to business will be increased.

However, I've not included in the budget all that I would like or that I think we need. Given the conflict between funding, which is low, and the operational needs created by rapid growth, which are great, I've given funding considerations precedence. Thus, I have been able to recommend property tax rates be adopted at roll-back levels, but only by eliminating 36 existing County positions and funding some of our elected officials at amounts less than they have requested. The budget is ambitious, but extremely tight.

With the assistance and cooperation of all County agencies, the staff, and County Commissioners, we will be able to attain all of our goals and objectives for this new fiscal year.

Sincerely,

John L. Smith
County Administrator

The third and final accounting category consists of **Fiduciary Funds.** These are also referred to as **Trust and Agency Funds.** These funds account for assets held by a governmental unit in a trustee capacity or as an agent for individuals, private organizations, other governmental units, and/or other funds.

Examples: Confiscated Trust Fund
Inmate Trust Fund
Law Enforcement Trust Fund

Elements of a Budget Document

Despite wide differences in style, content, and amount of detail, budget documents usually consist of four basic elements, described here in detail:

1. **The Budget Message,** located in the front of the budget document, is the narrative that summarizes the fiscal year's budget. The information contained in this section should summarize the government's fiscal and management plan for the upcoming fiscal year.

The budget message usually highlights the fiscal and political climate that sets the tone for the budget process, identifies new and/or expanded programs, discusses the service levels at which operations are funded, and identifies any major or significant changes in revenue sources and/or receipts. The chief executive, usually a mayor or manager, normally prepares and signs the message for submittal to the legislative body of elected officials such as a city council or county commission (See Exhibit 1-4).

2. **The Budget Summary Data,** normally following the budget message, is the second element of the budget document. It includes several schedules of budget data. The number and type of schedules will vary with each local government's legal requirements, organizational structure, and elected officials' data preference.

Budget Summary schedules commonly used in a budget document include Millage Rate/Property Tax Information (Exhibit 1-5), Summary of Revenues and Expenditures (Exhibit 1-6), Revenues By Source (Exhibit 1-7), Expenditures By Fund (Exhibit 1-8), and Expenditures By Program (Exhibit 1-9). We will discuss each in some detail:

Millage Rate/Property Tax Information is important becase it identifies the taxable value of property upon which the local government can levy its millage rate(s). Property tax collections are the single largest source of revenue for most local government jurisdictions, therefore it is useful to understand how property tax collections are determined.

Exhibit 1-5 contains all the information required to compute this local government's property tax collections. The general formula for computing tax collections is as follows:

$$\frac{\text{Taxable valuation x adopted millage rate(s)}}{1000} = \text{Property Tax Collections}$$

Exhibit 1-5   Millage Rate / Property Tax Information

Tax Levy	FY 1987-88 Budgeted	FY 1986-87 Budgeted
General Fund	$43,325,496	$41,282,000
Capital Improvement Fund	4,638,834	4,418,646
Hospital Bonds	163,129	275,429
Library	2,568,890	2,445,023
Unincorporated Area MSTU	2,968,771	2,827,200

FY 1986-87 Taxable Value =	$11,296,399,080
New Construction =	577,015,690
FY 1987-88 Taxable Value =	$11,873,414,770

Budgeted tax amounts are 95% of the total property tax revenues levied due to anticipated uncollectible or delinquent taxes.

	FY1984-85	FY1985-86	FY1986-87	FY1987-88 Budget
General Fund	3.844	3.994	4.043	3.841
Capital Improvement Fund	.555	.427	.433	.411
Hospital Bonds	.029	.024	.027	.014
Library	.175	.197	.257	.243
Unincorporated Area MSTU	.461	.440	.445	.416

It should be noted that local governments often budget tax collections at 95%. This provides a cushion in the event that the collection of taxes is not 100%. Thus, in Exhibit 1-5, property tax collections for the General Fund are computed as

$$\$11,873,414.770 \times 3.841/1000 \times 95\% = \$43,325,496$$

This exhibit also provides the reader with the millage rate history for the local government. One can see that there have been millage rate decreases for the FY 1987-88 budget year from the prior fiscal year for each of the five funds listed.

A more detailed look at the property tax is contained in Chapter 7.

Summary of Revenues and Expenditures provides the reader with a condensed version of the governmental entity's budget. It identifies the major revenue sources, as well as the expenditure (cost) categories to which the dollars will be allocated. Exhibit 1-6 displays this data for four of a local government's many funds.

In reviewing the information contained in Exhibit 1-6, one can note that Taxes are the main source of revenue for all the funds identified, that Personal Services is usually the cost category receiving the major portion of monies allocated for disbursement, and that projected revenues equal

Exhibit 1-6 Revenue and Expenditure Summary

	General	Hospital District	Municipal Service District	Library
REVENUES				
Taxes	$40,069,108	$1,740,000	$ 6,500,200	$3,823,521
Licenses and Permits	75,000	0	0	0
Intergov't Revenues	6,218,285	0	5,082,500	269,409
Charges for Services	8,360,711	0	621,000	24,000
Fines and Forfeiture	1,160,000	0	0	50,000
Miscellaneous Revenues	839,000	60,000	498,000	70,200
Non-Revenues	4,209,355	0	5,035,000	376,022
Total Revenues	60,931,459	1,800,000	17,736,700	4,613,152
EXPENDITURES				
Personal Services	$30,308,170	$ 0	$ 5,627,291	$2,394,982
Operating Expenses	19,053,152	1,000,000	4,392,332	1,645,547
Capital Outlay	1,740,597	0	1,633,498	185,123
Sub-Total Operating	51,101,919	1,000,000	11,653,121	4,225,652
Capital Improvements	210,057	800,000	5,915,000	0
Debt Service	300,068	0	0	0
Grants and Aids	5,195,029	0	0	0
Transfers	2,701,574	0	0	25,500
Reserves	1,422,812	0	168,579	362,000
Total Expenditures	60,931,459	1,800,000	17,736,700	4,613,152

Exhibit 1-7 Revenues by Source

Taxes	$ 56,249,959
Licenses and Permits	2,032,000
Intergovernmental Revenues	20,236,320
Charges For Services	29,764,030
Fines and Forfeitures	2,580,000
Miscellaneous Revenues	4,504,225
Non-Revenues	
Contributions	1,132,104
Loan Proceeds	886,534
Bonds	7,200,000
Transfer From Other Funds	12,101,242
Appropriated Fund Balances	18,709,120
Total Revenues	$ 155,395,534

expenditures in each fund because local governments must balance their budgets. It is common in all governmental jurisdictions for Personal Services to comprise more than 50% of an agency's budget.

Revenues By Source information provided in Exhibit 1-7 enables the reader to identify the major sources of revenue for a different local government. Once again, one can see that Taxes are the primary revenue source. In this exhibit, the next largest revenue source is that of Non-Revenues. This category is comprised of loan proceeds, bond issue receipts, transfer of monies from other funds, and appropriated fund balances. (Appropriated fund balances are the monies not expended in the prior fiscal year and are appropriated to the next fiscal year's budget.)

Other sources which generate revenues for governmental units are Charges for Services (recreation fees, waters sales), Licenses and Permits (occupational licenses, building permits), Fines and Forfeitures (monies received from traffic tickets, beach fines, etc.), and Intergovernmental Revenues (local, state, and federal grants and revenue-sharing dollars).

Exhibit 1-8   Expenditures by Fund

	Actual FY 85-86	Current FY 86-87	Budget FY 87-88
General			
Council and Manager	$ 1,397,880	$ 1,672,240	$ 1,822,347
Public Works	260,186	306,847	339,351
Public Services	4,639,984	5,436,367	1,377,265
Public Safety	8,269,609	10,540,168	10,156,601
Finance	3,889,027	4,656,998	4,957,120
Corrections	8,481,635	10,260,159	11,483,390
Judicial	3,371,315	4,220,237	5,131,755
Community Services	1,141,044	2,289,282	2,612,699
Public Health Services	- - - - -	- - - - -	1,984,470
Planning and Zoning	684,685	1,210,370	1,644,851
Beach Management	- - - - -	- - - - -	5,460,529
Elections	1,028,156	935,055	1,140,368
Assessments	2,333,933	2,624,934	2,823,222
Agriculture	306,199	394,204	366,450
Total General	$ 35,803,653	$ 44,546,861	$ 51,300,418
Voted Gas Tax			
Public Works	$ 2,040,244	$ 2,095,597	$ 2,050,500
Library			
Public Services	$ 2,849,602	$ 3,275,258	$ 3,885,173
Advertising Tax District			
Tourist Development	$ 52,092	$ - - - - -	$ - - - - -
Criminal Justice Training			
Corrections	$ - - - - -	$ 162,911	$ 215,711
Public Safety	- - - - -	201,696	219,096
Total CJ Training	$ - - - - -	$ 364,607	$ 434,807

Expenditures By Fund is a schedule which details how monies are appropriated within each fund. Exhibit 1-8 displays actual expenditure information for several funds for the prior budget year (column no. 2), estimates for the current budget year (column no. 3), and planned spending for the budget year (column no. 4). Examples of fund titles are indicated by bold type in column no. 1.

In looking at the expenditure information provided for the Advertising Tax District, the reader can see that the fund existed in the fiscal year 1985-86, however there is no data for the "Current Year" or "Budget Year." This would lead one to conclude that the fund is no longer in existence. Likewise, in reviewing the expenditure information for the Criminal Justice Training Fund, one can see that this fund did not exist until fiscal year 1986-87. Apparently this is a new fund for the governmental entity.

This schedule is useful in that it contains important expenditure information for each fund. One can easily identify any major fluctuations in fund/departmental expenditures, as well as determine how long the fund/department has been in existence.

Expenditure By Program is the final schedule utilized by most governmental jurisdictions. This schedule details expenditures by major program categories (General Government, Public Safety, Leisure Services, etc.).

Exhibit 1-9   Expenditures by Program

General Government		Health and Human Services	
Assessments	$ 2,780,365	Agriculture	$ 399,652
Council and Manager	1,900,110	Community Services	3,064,569
Elections	1,924,934	Public Health Services	2,502,177
Finance	5,714,431	Total	$5,966,398
Total	$12,319,840		
Leisure Services		Economic Development	
Beach Management	$ 6,341,868	Ocean Center	$2,174,031
Ponce De Leon Port		Planning and Zoning	1,590,771
Authority	4,002,404	Total	$3,764,802
Public Services	6,149,886		
Total	$16,494,158		
Transportation		Environment	
Airport	$ 5,507,858	Environmental	
Votran	8,304,552	Management	$ 695,634
Total	$13,812,410		
Public Safety		Public Works	
Corrections	$14,501,683	Public Works	$39,969,531
Fire Services	4,744,619		
Judicial	5,977,069		
Public Safety	18,712,022		
Total	$43,935,393		
Debt Service		Utilities	
Debt Service	$ 9,127,875	Water and Sewer	
		Utilities	$9,309,493
Total Expenditures		$155,395,534	

By reviewing Exhibit 1-9, one can note that the Public Safety Program has been allocated the most money for expenditures. This is common in most governmental jurisdictions. It is also important to notice that the total program expenditures in Exhibit 1-9 also match the total revenue sources detailed in Exhibit 1-7, Revenues By Source. This is expected since local governments are required to adopt a balanced budget, unlike the Federal government which is accustomed to deficit spending.

3. **The Program/Departmental Data** section normally contains the budgetary and narrative expenditure information as related to the organization's structure. It is usually presented in one of the three budget types discussed earlier: line-item, program, or performance.

Exhibit 1-10 provides the reader with a departmental line-item budget format. The budget is composed of specific line items or object codes. This is a very detailed budget format and is a good mechanism for budgetary control and management of an organization's activities.

Exhibit 1-10   Sample Agency Line-item Budget

```
Agency:   Elections

Object                                    88-89 Budget
  Code      Item Description

Personal Services:

  1100      Salary - Executive          $    65,161
  1201      Salary - Regular                425,000
  1300      Salary - Temporary               15,600
  1400      Overtime                          6,000
  1501      Ed Incentive Pay                 19,000
  2100      FICA                             29,750
  2200      Retirement                       42,500
  2301      Insurance - Group                30,000
  2302      Insurance - Life                  4,250
  2400      Insurance - Work/Comp             8,935
  2500      Unemployment Insurance              400

            Total Personal Services     $   646,596

Operating Expenses:

  3400      Contracted Services         $    74,500
  3650      Janitor Services                  8,768
  3710      Data Processing Charges          50,000
  3810      Training                         10,170
  4000      Travel                           19,000
  4700      Printing                         19,000
  5100      Office Supplies                  50,000
  5420      Memberships                       1,000

            Total Operating Expenses    $   232,438

Capital Outlay:

  6410      Desk                        $       300

            Total Elections             $   879,334
```

Exhibit 1-11   Sample Agency Program Budget

Program: Leisure Services	Actual 1981-82	Adopted 1982-83	Revised 1982-83	Budget 1983-84
Administration	$16,522	$17,035	$21,342	$25,000
Playgrounds	14,896	15,140	15,140	16,000
Summer recreation	13,996	13,310	13,310	14,500
Cultural activities	3,551	3,170	5,120	6,000
Swimming	13,562	13,990	14,500	15,000
Community center	1,095	2,000	2,000	2,000
Parks maintenance	4,061	3,525	3,525	4,200
Beach facility	5,911	6,340	7,230	8,500
	$73,594	$74,510	$82,167	$85,800

Exhibit 1-11 would be described as a program budget format. The financial data is provided by major programs within the agency. Current year totals are shown in two ways: the original adopted budget for the fiscal year and later, revised budget figures adopted due to unanticipated expenditures thus far in the current year.

Exhibit 1-12 illustrates a performance-based budget. This format provides the reader with unit cost category information and enables one to understand how much it "costs" to perform a service.

The format that is utilized by local governments to present their financial/narrative information related to programs varies with each jurisdiction's need to emphasize control, planning, or management. However, any of the above described formats are suitable and will provide the reader with a good understanding of a government's budget. Each is widely used, often in combination with other formats.

4. **Supplemental Data Schedules** usually consist of additional information concerning the governmental entity, as well as any other pertinent data that does not fit appropriately into other sections of the document. Supplemental schedules that may appear in a budget document are:

- **Ordinances** that relate specifically to the local government's budget process

- **Capital Outlay and/or Capital Improvement Schedules**

- **Debt Service Schedules** that detail existing debt obligations

- **Glossary** that defines terms and concepts relevant to a budget/budget process/budget document

The areas cited above are not all-inclusive. The type of supplemental data included in a budget document is dependent upon the governmental entity's requirements.

Exhibit 1-12   Sample Agency Performance Budget

```
                        Expenditure Request Form
                          Department:  Fire
```

	Actual 1981–82	Current 1982–83	Budget 1983–84
Cost			
Fixed costs-administration	12,460	13,085	13,650
Fixed costs-fire prevention	24,085	27,825	29,295
Variable costs-fire companies	33,070	36,790	44,385
	$69,615	$77,700	$87,330
Manpower (Man-hours)			
Administration	4,160	4,160	4,160
Fire prevention unit	7,488	8,320	8,320
Fire companies	19,564	20,440	23,360
	$31,212	$32,920	$35,840
Inspections Performed (Number)			
Fire prevention unit	9,634	10,500	10,500
Fire companies	94,493	102,200	116,800
	$104,127	$112,700	$127,300
Unit Costs ($/Inspection)			
Fire prevention unit	2.50	2.65	2.79
Fire companies	.35	.36	.38

Notes on Calculations:

1)   Fixed costs-administration. Revised expenditure for the current year based on full staffing. Next year's estimate is also based on full staffing and 5 percent pay raise.

2)   Fixed costs-fire prevention unit. Uses the same estimating basis as administration.

3)   Variable costs-fire companies. Revised expenditures for the current year are based on the number of inspections to be delivered by the fire companies and paid for at the rate of 36 cents per inspection. Inspection rates are estimated at 38 cents per inspection for next year's expected work load of 116,800 company inspections.

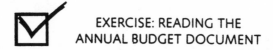

EXERCISE: READING THE
ANNUAL BUDGET DOCUMENT

If possible, obtain a copy of your local government's budget document and use it to answer the following questions. If this is not possible, use the exhibits in this chapter as the basis for your responses.

1. Read the Budget Message (Exhibit 1-4) and identify major points that the chief executive provides for the elected officials.

2. Refer to the "Millage Rates" portion of Exhibit 1-5. Provide a reasonable explanation as to why the Hospital Bonds millage rate decreases annually. Also, gather millage rate information related to your local city or county. Do the millage rates reflect any major increases in tax levys? What issues may have caused the need for such increases?

3. Look at the "Expenditures" section of Exhibit 1-6. For each fund group, calculate the percentage of the "Sub-Total Operating Expenses" represented by Personal Service costs. Do these percentages seem reasonable, too high, or too low? Also, what is the relationship between revenues and expenditures within each fund?

4. Review the information provided in Exhibits 1-8 and 1-9. Identify the programs that are the major spending areas. Explain why these areas require the most appropriation of funds.

5. Which budget format (line-item, program, or performance) do you find the most informative and beneficial? Justify your answer by reference to Exhibits 1-10, 1-11, and 1-12.

NOTES

1. Adapted from Edward A. Lehan, *Simplified Governmental Budgeting* (Chicago, Illinois: Municipal Finance Officers Association, 1981), p. 79.

2. "Number and Classification of Funds," in *How Your Government Can Apply GAAP* (Cleveland, Ohio: Ernst and Whinney, 1982), p. 54.

_____

Chapter 2

COPING WITH THE BUDGET PROCESS _____

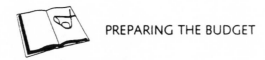 PREPARING THE BUDGET

HOW THIS CHAPTER WILL BE USEFUL

This book was written for current public managers and those who aspire to careers in government administration.

In the first chapter of this workbook, you learned to be an intelligent **consumer** of the annual government budget document for your jurisdiction. Now you should be able to seek (and find!) particular information in the budget and interpret the various tables, figures, and graphs. Most importantly, you should be able to interpret the implications the budget has for your community, your local government, your agency, and your own job responsibilities. You are already a far more capable budgeter than the vast majority of government employees!

However, as a public administration professional, you also need to know how the budget is created, and how you can be an effective **producer** in this budget creation process. Thus, the remainder of this book is devoted to helping you master the basic skills of preparing, winning approval for, and executing good agency budgets.

In this chapter, we intend to give you an overview of the process by which a budget is prepared to guide the operations of a local government. Although every jurisdiction has its own unique combination of legal constraints, historical customs, staff capabilities, formal procedures, and informal processes, the basic process remains about the same everywhere. This process is designed to produce, among other things, good agency budgets. By good agency budgets, we mean budgets which accomplish two important goals simultaneously:

- First, they provide a sound plan and adequate funding for the programs, objects, and activities which must be purchased for an agency to do its job in the coming fiscal year, and

Exhibit 2-1   The Budget Process

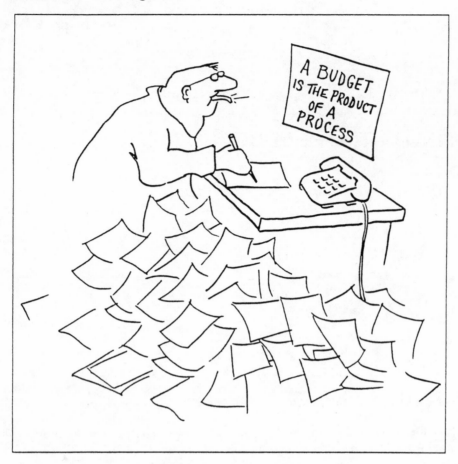

- Second, they recognize the fiscal situation and policy priorities of the larger jurisdiction of which the agency is a part.

OBJECTIVES

The purposes of this chapter are to enable you to:

1. Identify the four phases of the budget cycle.

2. List and describe the basic elements of the formal budget preparation process.

3. Explain the concepts and procedures involved in a rational management approach to budget development.

4. Explain the impact of the balanced budget requirement, political climate, and human limitations on local government budgets.

THE BUDGET PROCESS

The Phases of the Budget Cycle

In order to be effective in their local government's annual budget preparation process, public managers need to become familiar with the formal requirements of the system including calendars, forms, and various documents. In addition, they must be prepared to participate in developing and presenting their agency budget from both a highly rational, management-oriented perspective, and also from a more "real world" viewpoint which includes legal, political, and human limits on what can be done.

The first step in grasping the budget process is to learn the four phases of what is usually called "the budget cycle," including preparation, approval, execution, and audit.

1. **Preparation.** First, agencies prepare budget requests based upon their experiences of the past, their plans for the coming year, and guidelines received from the Chief Executive or administrative staff such as a Central Budget Office. Then, the executive and staff review and adjust the requests in light of available revenues, policy priorities, and political necessities. Finally, a recommended budget is assembled.

2. **Approval.** The recommended budget becomes a legally binding document only upon passage by the legislative body, such as a city council, county commission, or school board. Usually, at the local level, the executive's recommended budget survives the approval process relatively unchanged. This is in part due to the limited time and staff available to legislators. However, it is also in part a result of the executive anticipating the legislators' preferences regarding taxes and spending, including particular legislator's personal priority programs.

3: **Execution.** The adopted budget goes into effect with the beginning of the fiscal year. Since a budget is a plan based on estimates of future revenues and future expenditures, close monitoring of both income and spending is required in order to be prepared to make adjustments should revenues fall short of what has been anticipated or should special circumstances cause spending to exceed expectations. In any case, agencies must manage their budgets carefully to ensure that funds last through the fiscal year. Generally, the chief executive or central budget office will control the flow of funds to agencies through apportionments or allotments on a monthly or quarterly basis to assist in the process.

4. **Audit.** The final stage of the budget process is intended to guarantee that the budget execution phase was handled with honesty and in compliance with the legally adopted budget. Specific accounting procedures are followed and outside auditors check the books to accomplish this purpose. Over the years, the scope of auditing has expanded to include review of the efficiency and effectiveness of spending programs. While this trend is most pronounced at the federal and state levels of government, it is beginning to impact even small and middle sized local governments as well.

The budget execution phase takes the entire twelve months of the fiscal year to complete. This means that the budget preparation and approval stages must take place before the beginning of the fiscal year, while the audit phase necessarily comes afterwards. The larger and more complex the local

Exhibit 2-2   The Budget Cycle

```
                *   1989  *          1990                     *
                O   N  D  J  F  M  A  M  J  J  A  S  O  N  D  J

FY 1989    *    Audit    *

FY 1990    *          Execution                  *  Audit

FY 1991         *  Preparation  *  Approval   *  Execution
```

Local governments usually must work with two or three budget cycles
simultaneously, auditing the prior year, spending for the current year,
and preparing for the budget year (see Exhibit 1-1 for definitions).
In addition, most government fiscal years do not coincide with calendar
years. The calendar depicted here shows an October 1 through September
30 fiscal year. If today's date were November 10, 1989, the current
year budget would be known as FY 1990 even though it began in October
1989. In some parts of the country, the current year would be called
FY 1989-1990 to limit confusion.

[handwritten margin note: federal FY]

Exhibit 2-3   Budget Calendar Milestones

1. distribution of instructions and forms;
2. preparation of revenue estimates;
3. return of completed budget request forms;
4. completion of review and preliminary preparation
   work assigned to the central budget agency;
5. completion of executive review and executive
   determination of final budget content;
6. submission of the budget to the legislative body;
7. completion of public hearings;
8. preliminary legislative determination of the
   content of the appropriation ordinance or budget
   to be approved;
9. final action by the legislative body;
10. executive approval or veto of the adopted budget
    and legislative action;
11. completion of administrative actions, if any,
    needed to finalize budget appropriations;
12. beginning of the fiscal year.

government, the longer these phases take to complete. Thus, as Exhibit 2-2 demonstrates, public managers are often working simultaneously with budgets from three different fiscal years! Further, a significant amount of public spending is done for projects and programs which extend beyond a single fiscal year.

Finally, the fiscal year is usually structured to allow newly elected officials at least a little time to understand the budget process before they must plunge into decision making. Thus, the fiscal year rarely coincides with the calendar year, leading to additional confusion. Exhibit 2-2 displays an October 1 through September 30 fiscal year.

In the remainder of this chapter, we will focus on the budget preparation process, turning to budget review and approval in Chapter 5 and budget execution in Chapter 9. The audit phase is not a principal concern of most line and staff public administrators, so we will refer to it only as it impacts the other phases.

The Formal System

The process of preparing the executive budget for submission to the legislature is driven by the need to complete the process (including legislative adoption) prior to the beginning of the fiscal year. Deadlines are very significant in the local government budgeting process. Therefore, the central document is a budget calendar. Exhibit 2-3[1] depicts the type of milestones which may appear on such a calendar, and Exhibit 2-4 displays a sample calendar based on a fiscal year beginning October 1.

The first step in the process is the distribution of forms and data to guide agencies as they prepare initial budget requests. This distribution often is organized into a *Budget Manual* which explains in detail how to write and submit agency requests. This mass of material is given focus by a budget call letter or memo, highlighting critical elements of the preparation schedule and providing general policy guidelines for managers as they prepare their particular agency budgets. A Sample Budget Call Memo is included in Exhibit 2-5. As you can see, it alerts agency officials to the upcoming budget preparation procedures. Please note that:

- The first paragraph refers to the use of similar forms and instructions in past years (see Exhibit 2-6 for an example of various forms used). This points up a critical fact about the budget cycle . . . it repeats itself over and over. This permits the accumulation of knowledge, but it should also caution the public manager that it is important to conduct oneself through the process in any given year in a way that establishes harmonious long-term working relationships and a solid reputation for professionalism and accuracy.

- The second paragraph points to one of the critical problems caused by overlapping fiscal years. Budget preparation for next year takes place long before this year's budget is spent, meaning that one must base estimates of future budgetary requirements on current year estimates, rather than on complete historical data.

- The same paragraph refers to "carry-over funding," dollars which if not spent in the current year may be available for spending in the next fiscal year. This highlights a major area of contention between budget officials, who seek to limit spending insofar as possible, and agency managers, who view the adopted budget as theirs to spend this fiscal year.

- The following paragraph refers to "revenue estimates," and requests the assistance of agencies which do produce revenues in predicting income for the future. An increasing

Exhibit 2-4   A Budget Calendar

Budget formulation, adoption, and execution involves the year-round interaction of many people at various levels. The purpose of the process is to identify service needs, develop strategies for meeting these needs, and to develop detailed revenue and expenditure plans to carry out the strategic plans. As such, the budget process incorporates the following activities:

Date	Activity
January-February	Development of the budget manual and the design and printing of budget forms. Staff meetings with Commission members to determine priorities for the budget year.
March	Distribution of budget packages (including capital improvement program request form, goals and objectives form, and revenue projection form) to operating units and elected officials. County Administrator meets with Division Directors to communicate budget policies and priorities for the budget year.
April-May	Office of Management and Budget review and tabulation of operating budgets, review and tabulation of capital improvement projects, and review of revenue projections.
May 1	Statutory deadline for submission of budgets for Sheriff, Clerk of the Courts, Comptroller, and Supervisor of Elections.
May-June	Compilation of the budgets--operating and capital improvement.
June	Division budget hearings with the County Administrator and/or designated Assistant County Administrator.
July	Distribution of proposed budget to the Commission. Commission budget review worksessions.
July 31	Commission certifies proposed millage rates to the Property Appraiser.
September	Two public hearings on proposed budget and millage rates.
October 1	Implementation of the adopted budget.

emphasis on user fees by many local governments is making revenue estimating a more widely shared responsibility.

- The memo goes on to remind managers that it is their responsibility to request an adequate budget; if they do not make the case for funding, probably no one else will.

- However, this is followed by two crucial statements which signal the advent of a "bad" budget year in which few new programs or program expansions will be approved. First

Exhibit 2-5   A Sample Budget Call Memo

Ocean County

May 1, 1987

TO: All Department Heads

FROM: County Administrator

RE: Fiscal Year 1987-88 Budget Preparation

Enclosed are the budget instructions, forms, computer reports and other materials to be used in preparing your FY 1987-88 budget request. Most are similar to those used last year.

The time period April 1-15 will be for departments to review their current budgets and estimate expenditures for the entire year based on actual expenditures through the first six months. These estimates will form the basis for projecting the availability for carry-over funding. From April 15 through May 15, the departments will develop their budget requests for FY 1987-88. The budget staff will then review these requests and make initial budget recommendations prior to the Administrator's hearings which are scheduled the week of July 6. Please review the enclosed budget calendar for other important dates.

A form related to revenue projections will be distributed to those departments that have revenues directly associated with their programs. Please give estimates for both the current and next fiscal year.

Department heads are encouraged to prepare their budget requests at levels necessary to provide adequate services to the community. When possible, program expansions should be offset by other reductions.

As you know, a substantial imbalance between revenues and expenditures is projected for the General Fund in FY 1987-88. Should this necessitate reductions, your input is needed so recommendations can be made in program areas you feel have a lower priority in your department. As part of your transmittal memorandum, please indicate what reductions you would make in your programs, if the total General Fund budget for your department was 5% less than your current FY 1986-87 budget. In addition, please assess the impact of the reductions on services.

If you have any questions, please contact our office.

---

the memo indicates that recommendations for new spending should be paired with recommendations for cuts in other existing spending. Second, the memo asks for a specific set of cuts that the departments would make should the General Fund budget be 5% less than the current fiscal year.

In combination, these policy guidelines, instructions, and forms become the basis for preparing the annual budget. In Chapters 3, 4, and 5, we will take you step by step through the process of preparing these documents and defending your requests. First, let's consider budgeting from two contrasting perspectives.

Agency Needs: Building Budgets Rationally

One way for public managers to approach the budget preparation process is to take a direct, rational path based upon the tasks the agency is called upon to perform. Such a method begins with

Exhibit 2-6   Forms Used to Build the Budget

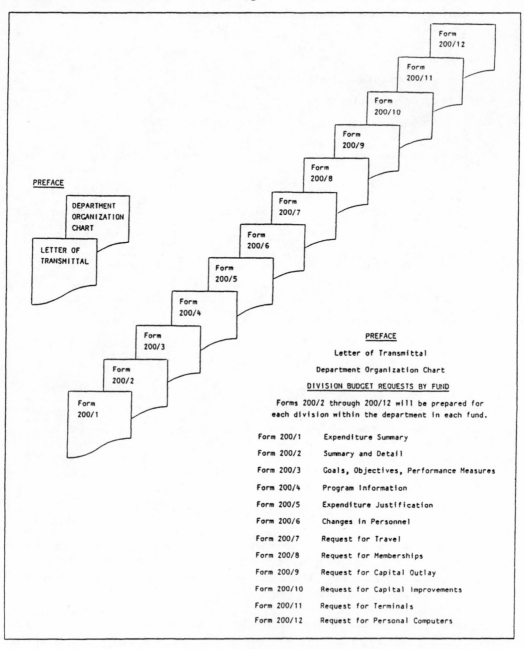

PREFACE

DEPARTMENT ORGANIZATION CHART

LETTER OF TRANSMITTAL

Form 200/1
Form 200/2
Form 200/3
Form 200/4
Form 200/5
Form 200/6
Form 200/7
Form 200/8
Form 200/9
Form 200/10
Form 200/11
Form 200/12

PREFACE

Letter of Transmittal

Department Organization Chart

DIVISION BUDGET REQUESTS BY FUND

Forms 200/2 through 200/12 will be prepared for each division within the department in each fund.

Form 200/1	Expenditure Summary
Form 200/2	Summary and Detail
Form 200/3	Goals, Objectives, Performance Measures
Form 200/4	Program Information
Form 200/5	Expenditure Justification
Form 200/6	Changes in Personnel
Form 200/7	Request for Travel
Form 200/8	Request for Memberships
Form 200/9	Request for Capital Outlay
Form 200/10	Request for Capital Improvements
Form 200/11	Request for Terminals
Form 200/12	Request for Personal Computers

the agency mission, which is derived from the legislation establishing the agency and is the most general statement of its reason for existence. As Exhibit 2-7[2] suggests, the mission statement is broken into increasingly specific goals and then objectives which express the criteria for successful agency actions. Basically, this is the notion of what is usually called "program budgeting." To the degree

24   PRACTICAL GOVERNMENT BUDGETING

Exhibit 2-7   Rational Path

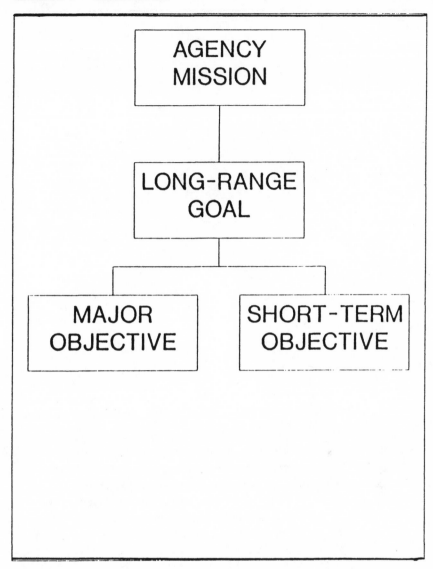

possible, objectives should be operationalized, meaning that their attainment can be measured at a reasonable cost. Goals and objectives may be relatively unchanged from year to year.

Once the objectives are established the agency managers must define agency output in terms of units of the services needed to obtain the objectives (see Exhibit 2–8).[3] This step brings us to what we have called "performance budgeting," by defining the quality and quantity of services to be provided. Finally, the resources needed to produce the particular level of service required to achieve the objectives must be specified. These resources then form the basis of a line-item budget request.

A simple example may clarify the method: The mission of a school system is to educate; one goal is to provide education to all children between the ages of 5 and 16; one objective may be to

Exhibit 2-8   From Objectives to Budget Requests

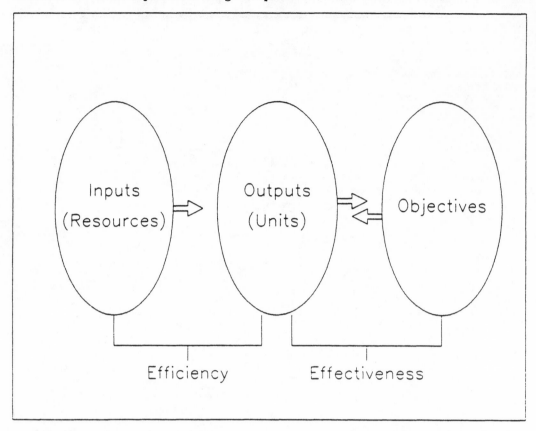

maximize school attendance of this age group. In order to maximize attendance, the school system might establish a procedure of attendance officer visits to the homes of absent children. The outputs of home visits in order to improve the measurable objective of increasing school attendance would require certain resources including an employee and transportation expenses to make the visits. If management were able to make reasonable estimates of the time and cost required for a typical home visit (efficiency) and the number of home visits to be made in the fiscal year, then the line-item budget requests for a certain number of personnel and related expenses could be calculated with considerable accuracy. When the impact of home visits on increasing school attendance (effectiveness) can be demonstrated, then the choice of a level of service (number of home visits) to be provided could be made with full knowledge of the relationship between costs and benefits.

None of this is necessarily very easy. However, efforts over a series of years to improve the clarity of objectives, to measure the units of outputs, and to assess the true and complete cost of resources needed can often lead to surprisingly solid information on which to base budget requests. In the next three chapters, you will learn how to perform these techniques.

External Impacts on Agency Budgets

If the budget calendar is the dominant feature of the budget preparation process, the legal requirement that local government budgets be balanced is the major force in the substance of budget preparation. Most agencies do not focus on this because:

Exhibit 2-9   The Popularity of Analysis

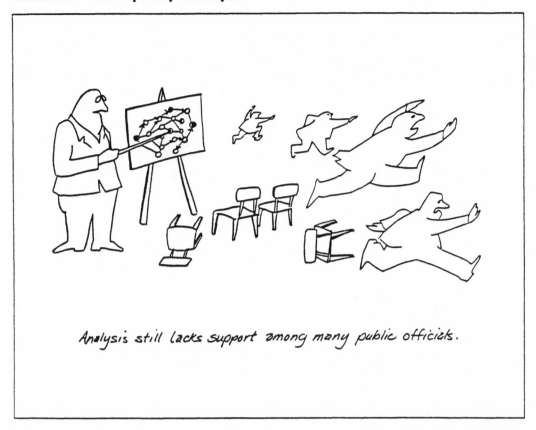

Analysis still lacks support among many public officials.

Agencies prosper—and their personnel prosper—when clients are pleased, and clients are pleased when favorable programs are operational or forthcoming. Since agency personnel do not have any responsibility for collecting money, they do not worry about balanced budgets or fiscal probity but leave such worries to others. Agencies, however, are in constant contact with substantive problems needing solutions and clients desiring service.[4]

On the other hand, the central budget office and the chief executive do have to face the task of bringing the sum total of agency budget requests down to the level of anticipated revenues. This simple and understandable conflict sometimes leads to stereotyping budget officials as cold, arrogant, and negative (see Exhibit 2-10)[5] and on the other side, agency managers as free-spenders, seeking to acquire more than their share of resources.

Another factor external to agency operations which impacts agency budgets is the political climate. What are the prevailing sentiments on taxes? What issues are in the forefront of public attention? What are the personal priorities of elected officials, individually and collectively? How many citizens, clients, or organized groups favor maintenance or expansion of particular agency operations? Again, while public managers are expected to implement public policy in a rational and neutrally competent manner, they can scarcely ignore the need to acquire resources or the corresponding need for political support in order to do so:

Exhibit 2-10   How Budget Officers Say "No"

Budget Office officials often are viewed as cold, arrogant, negative folks, simply because their jobs frequently require them to turn down requests which seem eminently reasonable to agency managers who make them. To avoid that unfortunate reputation as "the abominable no-men (and women)," good budget officers try to say things like:

o   "My hands are tied" - other factors may exist such as an executive mandate which precludes the favor.

o   "Maybe in the future" - the favor may be granted but the timing is simply not right.

o   "But look at the other positive actions we have taken" - stress that other decisions were in their favor and appeal to the notion that one should only expect to win a "fair share" of the time.

o   "It cannot be done" - economic, technical or other reasons can be cited to explain why the request is either impossible or extremely unwise to fulfill.

Since bureaus do not have exclusively economic outputs, their markets and consumers are most often clientele, organized interest groups, and political elites. They engage in exchange relationships with these essential actors to achieve legitimacy and domain **as well as political support for budgetary allocations** (emphasis ours). Political exchange dominates a bureau's market or environmental transactions and the evaluation or response to bureau outputs is political.[6]

A third external force impacting on the budget preparation process are the collective human and technical limitations of time, resources, and capability to produce the budget before the start of the fiscal year. The result is that a significant part of the budgeting process is the search for time- and labor-saving shortcuts to help complete the work and meet deadlines with minimal sacrifices to the quality of the final product.

A prime example of this is **incrementalism,** a process in which it is assumed that last year's spending provides an appropriate "base" for this year's spending. This assumption may allow some bad programs to continue, but it also permits all participants in the process to concentrate their efforts on requests for new spending, which probably deserve more scrutiny in any event.

An elaborated version of this perspective is presented in Exhibit 2-11[7]. Here the annual budget is viewed not as principally resulting from either rational planning or horse-trading political maneuvers. Rather, the budget is viewed as the product of a number of concessions to the constraints of the real world of limited capabilities. Thus, an agency budget is said to be the sum of last year's budget plus across-the-board increases in personnel costs, plus across-the-board increases for other costs due to inflation, plus the cost of expanding or extending existing services (if any are approved), plus the cost of new programs (if any are approved). For a lot of local governments, this is a pretty fair description of what goes on at budget time.

Unfortunately, this kind of approach to budgeting does not meet a professional manager's responsibilities to be an effective and efficient administrator of an agency mission and its services. This

Exhibit 2-11   The Incremental Budget Process

```
Despite the increasing sophistication of professional budgeting practices
in local governments, many believe that the true budget process, hidden from
view, goes something like this:

   o    Last year's appropriation, plus

   o    Automatic increases for existing personnel, plus

   o    Cost of inflation to continue existing level of services, plus

   o    Cost of additional service by unit (if any), plus

   o    New program costs or "quality" improvements (if any)
```

approach also fails to produce a budget document responsive and accountable to the taxing, spending, and policy priorities of the citizens. Therefore, public administration professionals should work toward a budget process which permits informed choices concerning the inevitable trade-offs between operating agency needs and overall government fiscal and policy priorities.

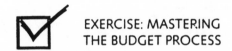

EXERCISE: MASTERING THE BUDGET PROCESS

In order to get a better feel for the budget process, the following simple exercise is designed to help you experience the processes and perspectives involved in government budgeting. Before you begin, please keep in mind two facts about this exercise:

- First, in the following chapters there will be exercises that will help you acquire or refine your skills in doing rather detailed budget work. For now, however, the exercise is simply to prepare what might be viewed as a "rough draft outline" for a budget request.

- Second, the exercise continues with a structured "mini-role-play" in which participants will act in one or more of four roles. We are well aware of the over-simplifications built into these roles, and you should be as well.

Notwithstanding these two qualifications, this exercise will prove highly useful to those without much exposure to public budgeting and will offer some helpful reminders and insights to seasoned veterans of the budget process as well.

Step One: Homework

- Students who are employed in the public sector should obtain a copy of their agency's mission statement. This can usually be located in the Adopted Budget, an Annual Report, or perhaps in a Management Plan which guides operations. If you are not employed in government and/or do not have access and adequate background on any

Exhibit 2-12   Agency Budget Proposal Form

```
                    Agency Budget Proposal Form

Agency Name:

Proposal Name:

Submitted by:                        Date:
_____
Need:




_____
Description:




_____
First Year Cost:

            Personal Services:
            Operating Expenses:
            Capital Outlay:
_____
Future Year Cost:

            FY 2:
            FY 3:
            FY 4:
            FY 5:
_____
Measure of Success:




_____
Required Changes:



```

---

particular agency, please choose from the options provided at the end of this chapter as Exhibits 2-15, 2-16, and 2-17.

- Now, keeping in mind the mission and your knowledge of the agency, identify one change (a new program or significant modification of an existing program) which you

Exhibit 2-13   Four Roles in the Budget Process

Agency Director: As the person with final responsibility for development and presentation of the budget request for your agency, your principal concern is to acquire the dollars necessary to produce the services your agency will be expected to deliver in the coming year. In addition, your professionalism, your loyalty to "your" people (employees, clients, or both), and your selfish interests all coincide in the desire to expand the quantity and increase the quality of those services.

On the other hand, you expect to continue in your position for years to come or be promoted. Thus, you want to be known as a team player, and would prefer to be thought of as someone with a perspective which extends beyond the limits of your agency.

Budget Officer: Your job is to help the Chief Executive evaluate and assemble agency budget requests into a single document which meets the needs of the Chief Executive, conforms to all legal requirements, is prepared on time, uses the proper format and codes, is mathematically accurate, can be defended in terms of agency mission-program objectives-performance standards, and does not waste taxpayers' money, particularly when there are many reasonable but unfunded requests for which the money could be spent. Your job is to determine a recommendation on the agency director's request and then defend your recommendation to the Chief Executive.

Chief Executive: You are the one official, whether elected or appointed, who is individually responsible for managing the entire local government for the benefit of all the citizens. You want a budget which: balances revenues and expenditures, keeps taxes down, provides agencies with the dollars they need to be effective service providers, reflects your own policy priorities, and will be adopted with minimal fuss by the legislators.

Legislator: Your position is part-time, low-paid, and full of aggravation. Still, being a legislator carries a certain amount of power and prestige, offers a chance to make a difference in your community, and may be of help in promoting your small business. You've been reelected once pretty easily, but you are always afraid that some big flap will result in real opposition. You don't want to get beat, but while in office you **are** going to express your opinions!

believe would improve the agency's ability to perform its mission. The total first year budget for your proposal cannot exceed $100,000.

- Using only the form provided *without attachments* (see Exhibit 2-12), please address the following:

1. Demonstrate the need for your proposal to be adopted.

2. Explain how the program would function when implemented.

3. Estimate the first-year cost of adopting the proposal. Note only three subtotals (personnel, operating, and capital outlay) and remember your first-year cost cannot exceed $100,000.

4. Estimate the annual cost for years two through five should the proposal be accepted.

5. Identify the best quantitative measure of program success or failure.

6. List changes (if any) which would be required at your agency in order that the proposed program be implemented.

Exhibit 2-14   Evaluating the Budget Role Play

An Assessment of the Budget Process Exercise

Student Name: Date:

_____

Did the role play(s) you participated in produce a "good" budget outcome
balancing agency needs and government-wide priorities?

_____

How did your proposal fare? Why did it succeed beyond your dreams, or, what
could you do to make it even more successful if you could try again?

_____

Pick three adjectives which best describe the budget process role play(s)
you participated in and explain your choices.

- Be prepared to make a two-minute oral presentation of your proposal and to answer
  questions from executive/budget officials and/or legislators.

- Bring at least two extra copies of your proposal to class to present for analysis.

Step Two: Role Play

- In class, your instructor will assign you to groups of four and to one of the following four roles: agency director, budget officer, chief executive, or legislator (see Exhibit 2-13 for details of each role). You should try to play your role as described, but feel free to be yourself within those limits. For instance, the legislator role description includes "you have your own opinions on spending priorities." If you play that role, please include your personal priorities as part of the legislator's behavior. If time allows, it is useful for each student to have a chance to play each role, ideally in a different group of students for each enactment. At a minimum, each student should have a chance to be agency director and present the proposal prepared as homework.

- Each agency director should meet with the assigned budget officer. The purpose of these ten-minute sessions is for the budget officer to determine a recommendation on the agency director's proposal for a program change.

- Meanwhile, the legislator and executive should get together to discuss the economic and public-opinion climate in regards to the upcoming budget hearings or just socialize with one another.

- Next, budget officers will discuss their recommendation with the chief executive. Agency directors will be available and will participate if the chief executive wishes to have their input. The legislator continues to socialize, possibly with legislators from other groups. These five-minute sessions will conclude with the chief executive accepting or opposing the budget officer's recommendation regarding the proposal.

- Finally, the legislator will join the group and review the written proposal (if it is recommended by the chief executive) to determine whether it should be included in the adopted budget. Agency directors, budget officers, and chief executive will be available but will give information only when the legislator seeks specific facts from them. If the proposal is not recommended, then the agency director may raise the subject with the legislator in an informal way. The legislator may then choose to follow up and review the decision not to include the proposal in the budget. This session may last from one to ten minutes.

Step Three: Assessment

- Each student should fill out Exhibit 2-14 individually and without discussion. This is an important part of the learning process, and needs to be taken seriously. Your instructor may wish to collect the forms to help determine what you have learned from the exercise.

Options

The method described above is intended to be quick and simple, minimizing preparation time and complicated logistics, thus giving as many people as possible a chance to participate directly in as many roles as possible. It is really just a series of conversations!

An option which would better simulate the real budget process, albeit at the cost of turning many participants into observers for most of the role play, would be to have many agency directors, a budget officer for perhaps every five directors, a single chief executive, and a group of legislators who

Exhibit 2-15   Sample Agency Description #1

AGENCY: WATER & WASTEWATER

MISSION:

To protect the public health by providing for the efficient and cost-
effective collection, treatment, and disposal of solid waste and wastewater
and to ensure a safe, clean drinking water supply.

DESCRIPTION:

This department provides residential and commercial water and wastewater
utilities to over 75,000 customers in various areas of the County.
activities of this department include maintenance of the water utility
systems and wastewater treatment facilities, engineering and construction
management of capital improvements, laboratory analysis, fiscal support,
and administration.

GOALS & OBJECTIVES:

1)   To provide efficient utility systems which comply with regulatory
     requirements and meet environmental needs.

-    Build, improve, and maintain a water utility system.
-    Build, improve, and maintain wastewater treatment facilities.
-    Maintain in-house engineering expertise and construction management
     for capital projects.

2)   To ensure that the utility systems protect the public health and
     environment.

-    Monitor water quality and wastewater effluent.
-    Provide quality assurance data to intergovernmental regulatory
     agencies.

3)   To provide trained personnel at all levels for effective operations.

-    Maintain a training program to ensure that personnel are knowledgeable
     in current technology.

PERFORMANCE:

Performance will be measured by the number of gallons of potable water
provided, number of gallons of wastewater treated, number of laboratory
analyses performed, number of customers billed, and number of training
sessions attended.

---

would meet jointly to consider all proposals recommended or brought to their attention through "off-the-record" means.

Another popular option is to bring in a city manager, municipal legislator, and/or local budget officials to review proposals from the students, who all play agency directors.

Exhibit 2-16   Sample Agency Description #2

AGENCY: OFFICE OF MANAGEMENT AND BUDGET

MISSION:

To utilize sound budgeting and financial reporting practices in accordance
with generally accepted accounting principles and conformance to standards
that would qualify the county for the Award for Distinguished Budget
Presentation and the Certificate of Achievement for Financial Reporting
from the Government Finance Officers' Association of the United States and
Canada.

DESCRIPTION:

The Office of Management and Budget is responsible for the preparation and
monitoring of the annual County budget and special projects as assigned by
the County Administrator's Office and the Orange County Commission. This
department coordinates and monitors all purchasing, financial, and personnel
operations throughout the year, as well as conducts management audits,
provides contracts administration and capital programming.

GOALS & OBJECTIVES:

1)   To develop a method of projecting future fiscal needs for the County.

-    Develop a fiscal trend monitoring process within the current fiscal
     year.
-    Improve the five year capital improvements reporting by requiring
     better reporting by Departments for the fourth and fifth years.

2)   To assure the citizens of the County that their tax dollars are being
     utilized in the most effective methods.

-    Develop and recommend an improved budget policy and a debt management
     policy.

PERFORMANCE:

Performance will be measured by the number of management studies performed,
departments visited, training sessions held, and standard procedures
developed.

NOTES

1. Thomas D. Lynch, *Public Budgeting in America*, 2nd edition (Englewood Cliffs, New Jersey: Prentice-Hall, 1985), p. 106.

2. Peter C. Sarant, *Zero-Base Budgeting in the Public Sector* (Reading, Massachusetss: Addison-Wesley, 1978), p. 34.

3. Ibid., p. 40.

4. John Wanat, *Introduction to Budgeting* (North Scituate, Massachusetts: Duxbury Press, 1978), p. 58.

Exhibit 2-17   Sample Agency Description #3

```
AGENCY:  HIGHWAY MAINTENANCE


MISSION:

To complete, and maintain a comprehensive road network to provide a safe
and  efficient means of travel to serve the needs of the County Citizens
and  visitors.


DESCRIPTION:

This department provides maintenance for the road and drainage systems
located  in the unincorporated areas of the County to include secondary
road  maintenance and construction of residential streets, maintenance on
the secondary drainage system, and maintenance to retention ponds.


GOALS & OBJECTIVES:

1)  To provide safe road surfaces and clean rights-of-way for all County
    maintained roads.

-   Maintain an inventory of pavement conditions to enhance response to
    complaints for repairs.
-   Schedule resurfacing on a fifteen year cycle.
-   Reduce water erosion of roadbed by installation of underdrains and
    full utilization of a pipe sealing crew.
-   Maintain a schedule of street cleaning in all districts.
-   Increase mowing and ditch cleaning schedule.

2)  To provide routine cleaning on County maintained retention ponds.

-   Maintain a schedule of cleaning five times annually for a projected
    number of 432 ponds.


PERFORMANCE:

Performance will be measured by number of miles of roadway resurfaced and
constructed, number of feet of drainage structures maintained, number of
miles  of streets and ditches cleaned, and number of retention ponds
cleaned.
```

5. Lynch, *op. cit.*, p. 89.

6. Harold Gortner *et al., Organization Theory* (Chicago, Illinois: Dorsey Press, 1987), p. 33.

7. Fred A. Kramer, *Contemporary Approaches to Budgeting* (Cambridge, Massachusetts: Winthrop, 1979), p. 8.

Chapter 3

BUDGETING FOR PERSONAL SERVICES _____

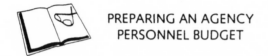

PREPARING AN AGENCY
PERSONNEL BUDGET

HOW THIS CHAPTER WILL BE USEFUL

The first two chapters of this workbook have familiarized you with how to read a budget document, as well as informed you on how budget preparation works. Now that you have a general sense of the budget process, the next major step is to learn how agencies actually prepare and submit their budget to the chief executive and the central administrative staff, such as the Central Budget Office, for review.

An agency's budget proposal normally consists of three main components or categories: personal services, operating expenses, and capital outlay/capital improvements (see Exhibit 3-1). Personal services includes costs for salaries and fringe benefits for employees, while operating expenses are comprised of costs related to an agency's ongoing operations. Expenditures in this category would include office/computer supplies, utilities, printing, memberships, tools and implements, contracted services, and any other items that relate to the "cost of doing business." Capital outlay includes items such as furniture, office equipment, and vehicles while capital improvements include costs related to projects such as building renovations, construction, and land acquisition.

This chapter is designed to assist you in preparing the personal services category of the budget. Accurate estimates for this portion of the budget are extremely important since personal services are usually the largest single element in an agency budget. Most agencies today utilize a computerized salary projection report in estimating personal service costs for the new fiscal year. This certainly makes the agency's task of projecting its employee salaries and fringe benefits much easier and faster. However, it is still beneficial to understand the mechanics of estimating personal service costs.

Exhibit 3-1   A Sample Agency Budget

```
        This sample agency budget shows the three main budget categories and
    subcategories of each. Note that Personal Services comprises by far the
    largest portion of the budget, which is typical of many "labor-intensive"
    government functions.

    Fund: General    Agency: Beach Management    Organization: Administration

    Object Code            Item                            Adopted Budget

       1201           Salaries                             $137,000

       2100           FICA                                   10,288

       2200           Retirement                             18,331

       2301           Group Insurance                         5,000
                          * Personal Services              $161,619

       3400           Contracted services               $    5,000

       4000           Travel and Training                     1,000

       4300           Utilities                               2,400

       4700           Printing                                1,500

       5100           Office Supplies                         1,700

       5220           Fuel/Oil                               10,000

       5420           Memberships                               500
                          * Operating Expenses            $     22,100

       6410           Office Equipment                  $      550

       6420           Vehicles                               10,000
                          * Capital Outlay               $     10,550


                       Total Agency Budget               $    194,269
```

This chapter will provide you with information that details those items that comprise the personal service category, as well as explain the techniques utilized in preparing a budget for personal service costs for existing employees and new personnel.

OBJECTIVES

This chapter will be useful in enabling you to:

1. List and describe the main elements of the personal services category.

2. Explain the steps involved in projecting personal service costs.

3. Explain the importance of providing accurate personal service projections in the budget.

PREPARING A BUDGET
FOR PERSONAL SERVICES

Importance of Personal Services

As explained earlier, a local government's budget is the most effective tool available for communicating its fiscal and management policies. The most important **and costly** element of this budget is that of personal services. Personal service costs normally comprise well over 50% of a government's budget. Unlike operating and capital expenditures, it is often difficult to curb or decrease personal service costs without implementing drastic means such as layoffs. The salaries of employees are an ongoing cost and they continue to grow annually. If a "budget imbalance" problem occurs in a local government's budget, you will rarely see an employee's base salary reduced or positions eliminated. Reduction in service level or the elimination of capital purchases are the first options considered when such budget problems arise.

There are also numerous fringe benefit costs that local governments must consider in preparing the personal service portion of the budget. One benefit, Social Security contributions (FICA), is required of all local government operations by Federal law. The percentage contribution is determined annually by the Federal government.

Other types of benefits such as group insurance, pension/retirement contributions, life insurance, or training supplements are usually provided by employers. These are benefits that the employer may not be required to provide but are additional forms of compensation for the employee.

Personal service costs are not completely precluded from consideration in reviewing expenditure requests. New personnel requests, proposed increases to fringe benefit rates, and pay plan adjustments are scrutinized closely as the local government tries to prepare a balanced budget.

Exhibit 3-2   Personal Services Terms and Concepts

---

o   **Cost of living adjustment (COLA)** - An annual monetary compensation awarded to all employees. The percent amount awarded is normally tied to the annual rate of inflation or the Consumer Price Index (CPI).

o   **Fringe Benefits** - Compensation that an employer contributes to its employees such as social security, retirement, life/health insurance, or training supplements. Fringe benefits can be either mandatory, such as social security contributions, or voluntary, such as retirement and health insurance benefits.

o   **Personal Services** - Those employee-related costs that include salaries and wages and fringe benefits.

o   **Salaries and Wages** - An employee's monetary compensation for employment.

The remainder of this chapter will cover position types, pay plans, budgeting for personal services for base/existing personnel, and preparing new personnel requests. A list of terms and concepts that are utilized with the personal services category is found in Exhibit 3-2.

Description of Position Types

Position types are important to budgets for personal services because they enable one to determine:

- The type and amount of fringe benefits that an employee will receive.
- The number of hours the employee will work on a weekly basis.
- The duration of the position.

The most commonly used position types are referred to as full-time, part-time, and temporary. Full-time (FT) positions are those that are scheduled to work on a full-time basis, normally 35-40 hours per week, and are eligible to receive full employee benefits. Part-time (PT) positions are scheduled to work less than the full-time positions, normally 15-20 hours per week, and generally receive prorated benefits. Library Aides or School Crossing Guards are often considered as part-time employees.

Temporary positions are designated for a specific period of time and may receive prorated benefits as well. Lifeguards who work during the peak season, i.e. April through September, or someone hired through a job service to fill a void while a position is vacant are examples of temporary positions.

A term often utilized by local governments in discussing numbers of positions is **full-time equivalent (FTE)**. This refers to the number of hours for which a position is budgeted. For example, a full-time position budgeted for an entire fiscal year would be the equivalent to 1.0 FTE, while three Lifeguards working full-time for six months would equate to 1.5 FTE's. By converting the number of positions to FTE's, local governments can view personnel in terms of **actual number of positions and their associated costs** needed to do the job and **not number of people**. This presents a more accurate picture of the size of the government staff.

Exhibit 3-3   Pay Plan by Class Title

Class Title	Class Code	Pay Range	Min	Max
Accountant	3330	B	17,654	26,334
Accounting Clerk	3305	107	10,362	15,546
Administrative Assistant	1012	D	21,405	31,961
Beach Ranger	3031	112	15,126	22,659
Buyer	1420	B	17,654	26,334
Clerk	1105	103	8,494	12,740

Pay Plans

Prior to preparing a budget for personal services, it is important to understand the local government's pay plan. The pay plan includes a listing of all position classes in the government and the minimum and maximum pay rate for each class. This is the means by which one determines how much salary an agency can pay for a specific position. Exhibit 3-3, Pay Plan By Class Title, includes the following information:

- Class Title—This identifies the title of the position.
- Class Code—This is a numerical identification assigned specifically to each class title. It is normally for use by the Personnel and Budget Departments only.
- Annual Salary—This column includes the minimum and maximum annual salary designated for each class title.

The pay plan is an instrument that is approved and adopted by the elected body of the local government and any changes to this instrument must be approved by the same body of officials. A well-constructed pay plan has a number of objectives[1], the most important of which are:

- To set salaries that are equitable in relation to the responsibility of work performed
- To make sure that rates do not discriminate against anyone
- To maintain a competitive position in the employment market, and thereby attract and retain competent employees
- **To provide data needed in budgeting, payroll administration, and other financial and personnel management activities**
- To provide an orderly program of salary policy and control

During the budget preparation process, agencies requesting new positions would refer to the pay plan in order to determine the pay rate allowable for a specific position. Also, in the event a position reclassification is requested, the pay plan would be consulted to determine what pay range for the reclassification would be most equitable when compared to positions of "like responsibility and duties" within the government organization.

Steps in Developing a Personal Services Budget

We will now describe the steps involved in preparing personal service budgets for base/existing personnel, as well as requests for new personnel. Prior to the budget preparation process, a manual is normally compiled by the Budget Office or administrative office designated with reviewing agency budget requests. This manual usually includes budget preparation forms, instructions as to how to complete the forms, cost information related to personnel, operating, and capital outlay items, as well as management policy information that agencies should consider when making their budget requests. Exhibit 3-4, Background for Salary Projections, and Exhibit 3-5, Fringe Benefit Information, are examples of instructions to an agency as to how the base/existing employee salaries and fringe benefits were calculated for the upcoming fiscal year.

Base/Existing Personnel Costs cover continuing employees. As stated earlier, most local governments today utilize a computerized salary projection report to determine personal service costs

Exhibit 3-4   Background for Salary Projections

```
The Salary Projection Report is to be used as a worksheet in preparing
salary projections for each division. A copy of this worksheet should be
submitted as part of the budget request package. The salary projections
are calculated for all authorized filled and vacant positions. Projections
for vacant part-time and seasonal (limited term) positions are based on
the minimum hourly rate for the job class and the number of man-years
currently authorized for those positions (i.e., 20 part-time positions =
10 full-time positions, therefore, each part-time position would be
scheduled for 35 hours per pay period at minimum hourly rate for position).

The salary projections include an average merit of 3%. The merit program
is currently under review by the County Manager's Office and the Personnel
Department therefore, this merit allocation is subject to change.
Departments will be contacted if any changes are made.
```

for base/existing employees for the next fiscal year. These reports automatically calculate each position's salary, as well as fringe benefits such as social security, retirement, and life/group insurance contributions. Salary is normally generated from existing payroll information while the calculations for fringe benefits are specific dollar amounts or percentages that are programmed into the salary projection program. (See fringe benefit information in Exhibit 3-5). These dollar amounts and/or percentages are applied to the employee's base salary in order to determine the total fringe benefit amount.

Exhibit 3-6 is an example of a computerized salary projection report. It provides the agency with all the basic information it needs regarding its employees and their personal service costs. Exhibits 3-4 and 3-5 provide a description for each of the items noted on Exhibit 3-6, Salary Projection Report.

The information contained in this report, and many local government reports, does not take into account any special compensations that may be required as the result of bargaining unit agreements. Items such as pay differentials for shift work, uniform allowances, or training supplements must be calculated separately. This information is normally supplied by the organization's Personnel Department.

Costs related to overtime payments or cost-of-living adjustments (COLA) are also calculated as separate items. Overtime is normally estimated based on prior year expenditures, as well as any potential increases in an agency's activity. The COLA is an annual adjustment approved by the local government's elected body and is provided to all employees. The rate of the COLA is often tied to the rate of inflation or the Consumer Price Index (CPI).

Merit increases are another form of compensation that are usually tied to an employee's annual performance evaluation. This compensation can be a flat dollar amount or a designated percentage amount that is determined by the legislative body.

With these exceptions, the data in the type of salary projection report shown in Exhibit 3-6 provides the basic information that an agency would need to project its base/existing employee personal service costs.

New Personnel Costs always receive special attention. As stated earlier, personnel costs comprise more than 50% of most local government budgets. These costs do not decrease each year, rather they are continually increasing. In addition, local governments try to keep the number of personnel to a minimum since the public has the conception that government has an overabundance

Exhibit 3-5   Fringe Benefit Information

Please use the information below to calculate the amount of employee fringe benefits to be budgeted per position:

FICA: 7.51% of the total salary up to $45,000.

Retirement: Calculated at 13.38% of the projected salary. Special risk positions are calculated at the rate of 15.35%. 17.43% of the projected salary for employees covered under elected state officer class and 6.15% of the projected salary for those employees who are reemployed retirees.

Health Insurance: Calculated at $1,273 per full-time person and $636 for part-time employees.

Exhibit 3-6   Computer Salary Projection Report

FY 1988-89   PAY PERIODS REMAINING- 26.1

FUND- 001 GEN FUND   AGENCY- Personnel

---------------P R O J E C T E D-----------------

Pos Title	Employee	Pay Level	Salary	FICA	Health	Retire-ment	Total
Clerk II	Jones, Ann	105	12,803.88	961.57	1,277.86	1,779.74	16,823.05
Director	Smith, Dan	9K0	52,732.18	3,439.58	1,277.86	7,329.77	64,779.34
Asst Dir	Wills, Jan	9G0	30,120.44	2,262.05	1,277.86	4,186.74	37,847.09

*Total salary determined by applying fringe benefit rates (Exhibit 3-5) to the base salary.

Exhibit 3-7   New Personnel Request Instructions

```
INSTRUCTIONS

Any requested change from current authorized positions should be reflected
on  this  form.   Please  distinguish  between  full-time  and  part-time
positions.

Use one (1) form per request

Section 1              Position:   Enter the position title requested.


Section 2              Number Requested:  Enter the number of positions
                       requested, as well as indicate whether the position
                       is full-time (FT) or part-time (PT).


Section 3              Pay Range:  Indicate the pay range.


Section 4              Personnel Costs:  Determine the base salary and
                       fringe benefits costs for the position and enter
                       in this section.  The Base Salary can be obtained
                       from the Pay Plan by Class Title Schedule (Exhibit
                       3-3) and fringe benefits can be obtained from
                       Fringe Benefits Information (Exhibit 3-5).


Section 5              Justification:  Provide written, detailed
                       justification for the new position.  Give
                       specific reasons and data that will provide
                       appropriate justification for the request.
```

of staff. Consequently, when new personnel requests are received, they are reviewed and scrutinized closely.

Any new personnel requests made during the budget process are usually submitted on a form that details the position request. See Exhibit 3-8 regarding New Personnel Requests as an example. This form requires three basic types of information:

- Position being requested accompanied by the costs associated with the position. Although not included in Exhibit 3-8, any associated operating and/or capital expenses which will be required for the new position should be considered.

- The number of positions requested.

- Justification for the position. This information is extremely important and must clearly address the need for the position.

These types of forms are usually accompanied by instructions (such as Exhibit 3-7), making the task of form completion easier for the user.

With these forms and data ready, it is now possible to pursue the various steps involved in preparing personal service costs for an agency budget. At the point an agency needs to estimate personnel costs, the decision has already been made as to the position classification, as well as the type of position (full-time, part-time, or temporary). **The first step** is to determine the pay range that has been designated for that position, as well as the annual salary for the position. In following the

Exhibit 3-8   New Personnel Request Form

Budget 19___   Agency Name _____   Account Number _____

| | | | | Personnel Cost | | | |
Position	Number Requested	Pay Range	Base Salary	Social Security	Retirement	Group Insurance	Total
Administrative Assistant	1-FT	D	$21,405	$1,608	$2,864	$1,273	$27,150

Justification:

Position is needed to handle the County's equal employment opportunity and affirmative action programs. The workload in these areas has increased 20% in the past year and current staff is unable to dedicate sufficient time required to handle these programs. New Florida Statute has created a significant impact on the workload in this area. Therefore, a new position is needed to expand, maintain, and administer these programs on a full-time basis.

---

example in Exhibit 3-8, we can look at the Pay Plan by Class Title (Exhibit 3-3) and see that an Administrative Assistant position is a pay range D with an annual salary of $21,405 to $31,961. Normally new positions are requested at the minimum of the salary range. In this case it would be the $21,405 as an annual salary which becomes the base for which all fringe benefit figures will be calculated.

The second step is to calculate fringe benefit costs associated with the position. In looking back at Exhibit 3-5 we can see that the following calculations need to be made:

- FICA - 7.51% of the total annual salary up to $45,000
- Retirement - 13.38% of the projected salary
- Group Insurance - $1,273 per position

All of the above percentages/dollar amounts are applied to the projected annual salary of $21,405 in order to determine the total fringe benefit costs for the position. (Refer to Exhibit 3-8 for the results of these calculations.)

The third step is probably the most important step in the process and that is the justification of the personnel request(s). The more information and statistical data that one can provide related to the need for the position, the better chance the position has of surviving the budget process. This written justification for the position must "sell" those who review the personnel request. If the justification is so poor that the reviewer does not even consider it after reading the information provided, then the request is "doomed to failure." **This personnel request should be prepared as if the agency will never have a chance to defend it orally** before the Central Budget Office, the Chief Executive, or Legislature.

These three steps should be repeated for each new position being requested. Understanding these steps and instructions should enable you to prepare a budget for personal services.

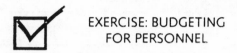 EXERCISE: BUDGETING FOR PERSONNEL

Using the following information concerning the Beach Management Department for fiscal year October 1, 1988 to September 30, 1989, please:

- Compute the full personal services costs for the entire Beach Department for fiscal year October 1, 1988-September 30, 1989. Separate costs into salary and fringe benefit components.

- Determine the cost to hire an additional Beach Ranger effective January 1, 1989 for the 1988-1989 fiscal year.

Personnel

POSITION CLASSIFICATION	ANNUAL SALARY PER POSITION	NUMBER OF POSITIONS	FTE
Beach Director	$47,000	1	1.0
Assistant Beach Director	35,000	1	1.0
Beach Ranger	20,000	10	10.0
Lifeguard	12,000	25	12.5
Secretary II	9,500	1	1.0

The county is part of a federal social security system. For the time period October 1, 1988 until the end of the calendar year, the county must pay 7.51% of all salaries up to $45,000 paid to an employee in the year. After January 1, 1989, the rate will increase to 8.0% on the first $45,000 of earnings.

The county pays a set amount of $1,250 per full-time employee for health insurance, and the amount is prorated for part-time employees. In addition, the county contributes .85% of each employee's annual salary for life insurance benefits.

Due to the seasonal nature of the beach, the Lifeguards are only on duty for the time period April through September, however, they are eligible for the same fringe benefits as the other Beach Department employees.

Beach Rangers also receive an additional compensation of $650 per year for attending training classes.

1. James Banovetz, ed., *Small Cities and Counties: A Guide to Managing Services* (Washington, D.C.: International City Management Association, 1984), p. 262.

Chapter 4

BUDGETING FOR OPERATING EXPENSES AND CAPITAL OUTLAY

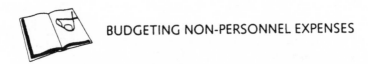

BUDGETING NON-PERSONNEL EXPENSES

HOW THIS CHAPTER WILL BE USEFUL

The budget process for local governments really begins with the development of agency budget requests. Public managers almost always have some responsibility for preparing or contributing to agency budget development.

Assuming an annual executive budget process, agency requests are proposed spending plans for the twelve months of the next fiscal year. These requests will be reviewed by the Central Budget Office, Chief Executive and Staff, and the legislative body. After final adoption, generally in modified form, the budget comes back to the agency as the legal authority to expend money for specified purposes in the fiscal year time period.

Ideally, agency proposals should reflect missions, goals, and objectives of the agency, as well as the judgement of the agency head with respect to scope, content, and quality of programs and activities that are being proposed to meet the agency's goals and objectives.

Budgets are submitted with a transmittal letter which highlights the agency's budget, identifying the objectives, program plans, performance expectations, and amounts requested to achieve the stated objectives (see Exhibit 4-1). The remainder of the request consists of data tables (which depict the spending plans in a variety of detailed and summary formats for decision-making purposes) and narrative statements (which relate expenditure plans to agency objectives and programs).

In the last chapter, you learned how to estimate personnel needs and prepare the budget documents necessary to fund the personal services for an agency. Here, you will learn how to prepare funding requests for the other two major categories in a local government's operating budget:

- **Operating Expenses** are the usual, ordinary, and incidental expenditures including contractual services, commodities and supplies of a consumable nature, current obligations, and fixed charges.

- **Capital Outlay** consists of equipment, fixtures, and other tangible property, the normal expected life of which is more than one year and the cost of which exceeds some set value (usually no more than a few hundred dollars). Land and buildings are considered **fixed capital improvements** and are generally treated as part of a capital improvement budget, separate from the operating budget we are considering here. (Chapter 8 covers the capital budgeting process.)

OBJECTIVES

The purposes of this chapter are to enable you to:

1. Prepare operating expense budgets utilizing a number of methods including incrementalism and unit costs analysis.

2. Prepare capital outlay requests with proper calculations and narrative explanations.

3. Demonstrate the use of such concepts as inflation, standard costs, continuing versus new versus improved programs, per capita service demand, and trend lines in preparing expenditure plans.

4. Explain the use of organizational units and object codes to build budget requests.

BUDGETING FOR EXPENSES AND EQUIPMENT

Budgeting For Operating Expenses

While personal services and equipment get close scrutiny in the budget process, other operating expenditures are generally neglected, except for a few items like travel and training which are too often assumed to be nonessential and targeted for cuts without close analysis.

The first building blocks of most budgets are established organizational units and object codes. On a day-to-day basis the government operates by organizational unit and must be held accountable on that basis. Thus, the burden for estimating expenditures during budget preparation normally rests upon the agency. The techniques used vary from the sophisticated to the arbitrary! Object codes enable effecive communication and control regarding those items the budget exists to purchase. (See Exhibit 4-2 for a sample object code format for operating expenses.)[1] The question is: how do we produce the spending estimate numbers for these operating costs . . . incrementally or based upon program and performance data?

Both of these general approaches make sense in many situations, and in fact, most local governments use some combination of the two. Here, we will first present the incremental method followed by three examples of analytical techniques: unit costs, predetermined charges, and standard costs.

Exhibit 4-1   Letter of Transmittal

Ocean County

June 15, 1991

Director
Budget Office
Ocean County

Dear Director:

Pursuant to State Statutes, County Ordinances, and the FY 1991-1992 Budget Planning Calendar issued by your office, enclosed is our Agency's requested budget proposal for FY 1991-1992. The information contained herein is a true and accurate presentation of our proposed work program for the next fiscal year. As Agency Director, I have reviewed and approved this submission.

In keeping with County policy regarding the upcoming year, our Agency has held requests for budget increases to an absolute minimum. However we are seeking:

o   Two new positions to process applications based on the approved workload standard per processor and the projected increase in applications, and

o   Increases in operating expenses to offset the unusual increases in supply costs faced by our Agency (justification enclosed).

We look forward to working with you towards approval of this budget request.

Sincerely,
Agency Director

The Incremental Method

In a strictly incremental, line-item approach, materials, supplies and equipment purchases are justified by detailed listings of the objects-of-expenditure and a comparison of these items to the previous year. A slightly more elaborate variation is to construct a trend line based on expenditures over the past few years and project it into the next fiscal year.

The line-item approach shows, for example, how many vehicles are to be bought, how much travel money will be spent, how much will go for printing, mimeographing, paper, typewriters, and stationery. The rationale for the specific dollar amounts requested is based upon agency spending in the past. While this is a clear and explicit type of budget, the method is probably best limited to small and difficult-to-estimate spending categories. Nevertheless, many jurisdictions use this approach as the sole method of estimating operating expenditures. Where the uncontrollable features of the future operating environment can reasonably be assumed to resemble the past *and* when we believe past practice reflects effective and efficient pursuit of agency objectives, this is a defensible method.

Exhibit 4-2   Object Codes for Expenditures

```
OPERATING EXPENSES.
Includes expenditures for goods and services which primarily benefit the
current period and are not defined as  personal services or capital outlays.

31.  Professional Services
Legal, medical, dental, engineering, architectural, appraisal, and other
services procured by the local unit as independent professional assistance.
Includes such financial services as bond rating, etc., where the service
received is not directly involved with accounting and/or auditing.  Also
include fees paid for competency and/or psychiatric evaluations and court
appointed attorneys.

32.  Accounting and Auditing
Generally includes all services received from independent certified public
accountants.

33.  Court Reporter Services
This includes the costs of appearance fees and transcript fees for in-court
proceedings, appeals, and depositions.

34.  Other Contractual Services
Custodial, janitorial, and other services procured independently by contract
or agreement with persons, firms, corporations, or other  governmental
units.

40.  Travel and Per Diem
This includes the costs of public transportation, motor pool charges,
reimbursements for use of private vehicles, per diem, meals, and incidental
travel expenses.

41.  Communication Services
Telephone, telegraph, or other communications.

52.  Operating Supplies
All types of supplies consumed in the conduct of operations.  This category
may include food, fuel, lubricants, chemicals, laboratory  supplies,
household items, institutional supplies, and uniforms and other clothing.
Also includes recording tapes and transcript production supplies.

53.  Road Materials and Supplies
Those  materials  and  supplies  used  exclusively  in  the  repair  and
reconstruction of roads and bridges.

54.  Books, Publications, Subscriptions, and Memberships
Include books, or sets of books if purchased by set, of unit value less
than $200 and not purchases for use by libraries, educational institutions,
and other institutions where books and publications constitute capital
outlay.  This object also includes subscriptions, memberships, professional
data costs, and training ad educational costs.
```

Even this method is not as simple as it seems at first glance. For instance, current year spending is in progress while the budget is being prepared, changes in the level of program quality or quantity may be planned, inflation may have affected the cost of items to be purchased, and efficiency improvements may be contemplated. These impacts should be separately calculated and, accompanied by narrative justifications, added to the base and across-the-board line-item adjustments if a purely incremental technique is used. We will learn to deal with these difficulties later in the chapter.

Exhibit 4-3 Operating Expense Report

Object Code	Item	Prior Year Actual	Current Year Estimate	Budget Year Request
34	Janitor	$1000	$2000	$7000
40	Travel	$1750	$3500	$5250
41	Phone	$3000	$6000	$9000
52	Paper	$ 450	$ 900	$1350

Exhibit 4-3 depicts a typical budget form used by agencies to request funds for operating expenses. It is patently obvious that the focal point of review and approval/disapproval of line items will begin with a comparison of the object of expenditure requests to past spending patterns. In all likelihood, only those items which depart significantly from past expenses will be given close scrutiny.

Several points can be noted from Exhibit 4-3. First, it seems that the budget request for phone, travel, and paper is based upon a very simple trend analysis in which the budget is expected to increase as much next year as it is apparently doing this year. However, costs for the janitor service contract are expected to increase significantly. Naturally, this item is likely to be singled out for justification. Finally, note that the impressively neat, organized, solid-looking figures above actually include only one column of hard data (and that is spending from **over a year ago**). Another column lists estimates for the current year's spending, probably based on six months or less of actual spending; and the third column represents what the agency hopes to get to spend next year. This simple illustration is pointed out here to emphasize that budgeters must not be mesmerized by tables of numbers. The assumptions, calculations, and analysis behind each set of numbers must be understood and, where appropriate, challenged!

Analytic Approaches

When budgeters go beyond the simplest kind of incremental or trend-line projections, they must realize that the techniques used should depend upon the type of expenditure. In any event, **judgement is more important than the blind application of some mathematical technique.** For instance, several factors should be kept in mind when ordering consumables:

- present inventory
- price levels including inflation and bulk order savings
- changing patterns in the use of materials
- changing requirements in relation to methods of producing results
- balance of materials to manpower so that manpower is not idle waiting for material

Exhibit 4-4   Examples of Unit Costs

Cost Center	Cost	Output	Unit Cost
Purchasing			
Processing	16,394	10,000 orders	1.64
Formal bidding	38,425	370 awards	103.85
Accounts Payable			
Vendors	63,490	33,600 payments	1.89
Employees	63,490	81,620 payments	.78
Accounts Receivable			
Taxes	74,303	37,000 accounts	2.01
Utility charges	20,082	225,000 payments	.08
Delinquent accounts	72,294	17,800 accounts	4.06
Tree Maintenance			
Trimming	90,266	7,500 trees	11.03
Removal	28,460	500 trees	56.92
Water Supply			
Well operations	515,075	25 wells	20,603.00
Well maintenance	222,151	25 wells	8,886.00
Ground Maintenance			
Playgrounds	68,355	38 sites	1,799.00

Every item requested should be examined using the same type of thinking: what information is available to help us determine what is truly needed and what it will cost? With this emphasis on judgement in mind, we now turn to three commonly used techniques for constructing agency operating expense budgets.

Unit Cost Calculations

At the other extreme of sophistication from incrementalism, agencies may use unit cost calculations to estimate operating expenses. **Unit costs** compare the volume of work anticipated to the items needed to complete the work and the funds required to purchase these items. This method can be used to justify the need for personnel or equipment, but its most common use in local government is in preparing budgets for operating supplies and services.

Exhibit 4-4[2] displays a number of examples of unit costs for various government activities and services, and Exhibit 4-5[3] displays a very complex system of data gathering developed to do the kind

Exhibit 4-5 Reports Used in Cost Accounting

Labor Reports: detail hours and type of work necessary to complete a particular task, project, or job.

Equipment Reports: note hours of use of each piece of equipment needed to perform a certain unit of work.

Reports of Work Done: measures volume of work accomplished.

Materials Reports: shows quantity and cost of all supplies used in producing completed work.

Invoices and Payrolls: include cost of supervision, utilities, space and any other overhead necessary for the work to be done.

Work and Cost Statements: compile various elements into comprehensive report on total cost of performing a given amount of work.

of cost accounting necessary to produce highly reliable statistics on which to estimate any kind of future spending, including operating expenses. Even simpler estimates of unit costs require considerable time and effort to develop, but can be highly useful at budget time for estimating the cost of continuing services provided at the same or increased quantities.

There are a number of disadvantages to using unit costs. These include: the cost of developing them, the fear that they can be used to cut what the agency sees as necessary slack, and the concern that quality and effectiveness will be sacrificed to quantity and efficiency if focus is narrowly on unit costs.

Predetermined Charges: Internal Service Funds

From the agency perspective, the easiest costs to calculate are those based upon costs determined or approved by the Budget Office. One good example is the charges of **internal service funds,** which support activities provided at cost to other departments. Common examples of local government internal service funds are:

- **Risk Management:** general liability and property insurance costs for the entire local government may be allocated to departments based upon their pro rata share of costs.

- **Central Equipment Pool:** maintenance of equipment can be provided with funding based upon monthly fees paid by each agency based upon its inventory of equipment.

- **Facility Management:** janitorial services and construction of building improvements may be billed to departments at hourly labor rates plus actual costs of materials

- **Data Processing:** provides services on a job rate charged to consuming departments.

- **Central Stores:** provides supplies to agencies at per unit costs calculated by cost of acquisition plus operating overhead.

- **Radio Communications:** maintains all radio equipment and charges for cost of labor and replacement parts at cost.

Exhibit 4-6   Standard Costs Per New Position

A standard expense and capital outlay package may be used to accompany requests for new positions. The expense package addresses professional and secretarial/clerical positions. The capital outlay package is based on current contract prices and addresses executive professional, technical professional, secretarial, and clerical positions. Any requests reflecting increases above these standards require justification. The following amounts are included in each package:

Operating Expenses

Item	Professional	Clerical/Secretarial
Telephone	$ 600	$ 450
Postage	100	75
Printing & Reprod.	100	100
Repair & Maint.	100	
Office Supplies	350	350
Building Rental	930	697
State Personnel Assessments	53	53
TOTAL	$ 2,233	$ 1,725

Capital Outlay

	Exec./ Profess.	Profess./ Technical	Secr.	Clerical
Desk, Exec. Sm.	302	302		302
Secretarial			430	
Chair,				
Exec. High Back	230			
Exec. Low Back		207		
Secretarial			125	125
Side Arm	260	130		
File Cabinet, 5 dr/w/lock	181	181	181	181
Bookcase, 6 tier	183			
Telephone, Rotary Dial	90	90	90	90
Calculator	186	186		186
Typewriter, Sel. III			661	
TOTAL	$1,432	$1,096	$1,487	$884

In some instances, the agency only needs to record the Internal Service "bills" assigned by the Central Budget Office. In other cases, staff may project the number of units of equipment to be purchased and multiply that figure by the assigned unit costs. Another option is to estimate the amount of labor to be utilized and multiply by the hourly rates.

Standard Costs

A final device for the determination of operating expenses is the use of standard costs based on ratios of expenses to well-known quantities such as numbers of employees or pieces of equipment. A **standard cost** has been defined as a forecast or predetermination of what costs should be under normal conditions, thus serving as a basis for cost control. All experienced managers and supervisors have informal standards which they consciously or subconsciously apply to their operations. These standards usually have been developed through years of experience. However, there is a tendency to judge entirely on the basis of one's own limited past experience and also to neglect the important factor of changing conditions.

Thus, Budget Offices try to develop more systematic approaches to the development of standard expenses in order to make the budget preparation process easier, control costs, and eliminate accidental or arbitrary differences in funding for the same items across agencies. In Exhibit 4-6, a sample package is displayed which identifies standard expenses to be budgeted for personnel when new positions are requested. For instance, office supplies for professionals are projected at $350 per year. Note that travel is **not** included in this example, requiring specific justification. Note also that agencies may seek increases in the package if they can provide adequate supporting data and explanations.

The rationale for these standard expense estimates may be based upon such factors as space standards, the complement of furniture for each position, the operating cost of a government vehicle per mile, the amount of miscellaneous supplies per position, the cost per square foot of maintaining buildings, estimated travel time and cost based on the number of travel days for each activity, the number of telephone units per 100 employees, or the printing and reproduction needs of each

Exhibit 4-7   The Politics of Equipment

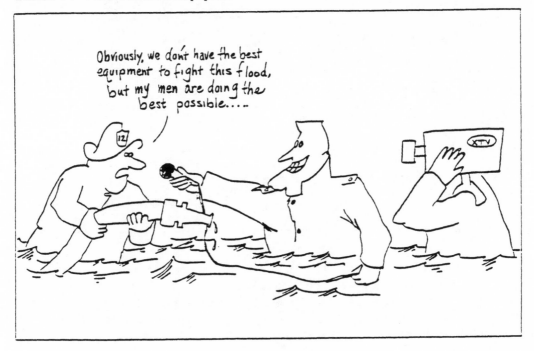

Exhibit 4-8 Capital Equipment Request Form

---

1. DESCRIPTION:_____

2. QUANTITY:

    Replacement:_____ Additional:_____ New Type:_____

3. ESTIMATED COST:

    Installed:_____ minus Trade:_____ equals Total:_____

4. SIMILAR EQUIPMENT ON HAND:

    _____

    _____

5. EXPECTED USE:

    Per day:_____ Per week:_____ Per month:_____

6. ADDITIONAL OPERATING COSTS:

    Personnel:_____ Supplies:_____

7. ITEMS TO BE RELACED:

    Make:_____ Age:_____ Maint. Cost:_____

    Planned Disposition:_____

8. MAINTENANCE COSTS:

    Anticipated Life:_____

    Annual Cost:_____ Total Cost:_____

9. BENEFITS OF NEW EQUIPMENT OVER PRESENT:

    _____

    _____

    _____

    _____

---

program and activity. To be effective, these standards must be prepared far in advance of the budget process based on cooperative research involving the operating agency, the central budget office, and the central supply or procurement agency. Once created, the criteria must be updated as work or cost conditions change.

Standard costs may also be used for "packages" of capital equipment. The Exhibit 4-6 example also includes the standard costs of furniture and equipment for new positions. These are, of course, capital outlay items, a subject of considerable frustration during the budget preparation process.

Capital Outlay

Equipment purchases often prove to be a problem for agencies seeking new or replacement items and for the Central Budget Office or other officials who have to review the wisdom of the agency recommendations. There are several reasons. First, equipment is usually considered easier to cut than personnel in hard budget times. Agencies may be asked why a copier machine is needed if they got by without it in the past, or why an aging typewriter cannot be repaired instead of replaced. Second, agencies frequently become enamored of the latest and greatest new tool with all the "bells and whistles" which will, in fact, make the agency more productive. Unfortunately, the true advantages of purchase may be hard to explain to budget reviewers pressured to find cuts in order to balance requested expenditures with projected revenues. **In short, budget battles over equipment are a classic case of "where you stand depends on where you sit." Budget balancers see frills, operating agencies see solutions to frustrations.**

Once an agency submits a capital equipment request (see Exhibit 4-8), there are four approaches to dealing with these conflicts between agencies and budget staff:

1. Use the standard cost approach, discussed earlier, which attempts to identify common equipment needs affecting many agencies and positions and to define quantitative standards of need. (For instance, one copier machine may be purchased per four secretarial positions.)

2. Focus on particular items. In the 1980s, the use of personal computers by professionals exploded. Many local governments established special procedures and review committees to develop and implement plans to computerize offices in a systematic and consistent manner.

3. Provide each agency with a fixed-ceiling amount for equipment expenditures and allow each to set its own internal priorities. This reduces conflict and gives agencies a "fair share," but the caps are inherently arbitrary since they precede any analysis of equipment needs across agencies.

4. Develop government-wide priority classification systems, as shown in Exhibit 4-9. This example, dealing with the purchase of motor vehicles, provides very simple priority guidelines for replacement based on age and mileage, allows for narrative justifications for exceptions to the criteria, and points out that the limited amount of funds available for vehicles for the entire local government necessitates the priority system.

In sum, **capital outlay budgeting is not a major calculation problem, it is a justification problem.** Estimating costs is usually as simple as volume-times-unit price. Predicting total equipment needs is often done for the agency by an imposed fixed dollar ceiling, but an open-ended approach

Exhibit 4-9   Vehicle Request Instructions

```
                         Ocean County
                    Fiscal Year 1991 - 1992
                      Vehicle Replacement
                     Policies and Procedures


Attached are instructions and submission forms for requesting new and
replacement vehicles. To take advantage of fleet discounts, specifications
for each type of vehicle have been established. However, selected options
may be justified operationally based on proposed use. Any request for a
variation not provided in this package will require exceptional
justification.

We can only fund manageable quantities of vehicles for acquisition next
fiscal year. Therefore, we will be utilizing the following replacement
criteria:



                              A        B        C

Trucks: Age (years)           6        5        4
Mileage (thousands)           70       60       50

Cars:   Age (years)           7        6        5
Mileage (thousands)           84       72       60


Vehicles in Category A will get serious consideration for replacement;
depending upon funding, vehicles in Categories B and C will get
consideration. Other replacement criteria such as the vehicle's performance,
maintenance and repair history, and the nature of its use can further
substantiate the need for a replacement meeting these guidelines.

New vehicle requests will be reviewed on the merits of the supplemental
justification, including need for the type of vehicle and its proposed use.

You should summarize your requests on the appropriate budget forms.
```

with government-wide priorities or reasoned review of each narrative justification is also used in some governments. If equipment replacement is planned, the equipment life is weighed by identifying the work to be done, the inventory, the service record, the procedures for inspection, and the quality of repairs done. If equipment additions are planned, careful consideration and justifications should be given to equipment use and equipment need. Capital outlay budgeting proves that budgeting should be more judgement than mathematics.

Some Special Considerations

Most local government budgets are constructed using year-to-year data comparisons accompanied by narrative justifications of exceptional increases or decreases for particular line items. Various program and performance measures, some more specific and quantitative than others, are usually relied upon to support these justifications. Special attention is given to anything that can be considered new spending. Continuing spending is regarded as part of the agency's base. Such programs have survived one or more years of budget scrutiny in the past and thus are presumed worthy of renewal except in unusual situations.

Exhibit 4-10   Changes Considered Part of Current Programs

Minor or technical adjustments to current operations

Deduction of nonrecurring expenditures

Adjusted cost to continue current positions

Price level increases/decreases

Replacement and most additional equipment

Adjustments for the continuation of electronic data processing costs

Annualization of current programs in order to reflect full-year funding for those programs initiated in the previous years

New positions and related costs due to increases in workload at the current level of services

Continuation of other personal services activities

Continuation of installment purchases

Continuation level for the nonrecurring appropriation categories

Fund shifts

Economies resulting from implementing cost effective measures

From this point of view, two considerations become absolutely critical to the accurate and effective presentation of a budget request. First, what should qualify as part of the agency's base spending? Second, what is the actual cost of continuing the past programs of the agency? To the unsophisticated, the answer to both of these questions may simply mean making a xerox copy of the current year's budget and changing the date at the top to the forthcoming fiscal year. In fact, answering these questions accurately and completely can make things considerably more complicated.

With regard to the first question, it is helpful to distinguish between proposed spending for current, improved, and new programs (also see Exhibit 4-10):

- **Current Program** is the continuation of services, functions, or activities now being provided, without a change in either the scope of the program or the standard or quality of the services, functions, and activities. Included may be price increases, new positions and related costs due to increase in workload at the current level of services, and increases to reflect annualization, which is full-year funding of programs initiated during the previous year.

- **Improved Programs** are implementation of changes in current operations that are intended to render services more efficient, economical, and/or beneficial. Efforts to improve the quality of services can also be included.

- **New Programs** are proposed services, functions, or activities which are not currently being provided and which are not part of any program now in existence, regardless of whether or not new legislation is required.

Exhibit 4-11   Inflation

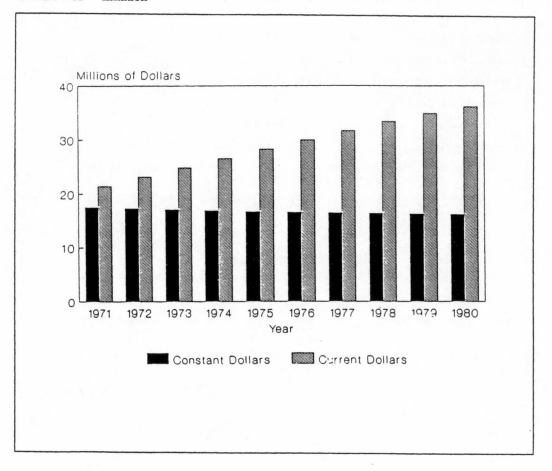

It should be obvious that the calculation of continuing program costs can be a highly complex endeavor. Further, the distinctions between new or improved activities versus continuing programs is hardly a cut-and-dried matter. **Working within the instructions of the particular jurisdiction, agencies must be certain to attribute continuing costs to their base budget** to avoid shortfalls in budget allocations which will cause unintended quality and/or quantity service cutbacks. New or improved programs should be presented as such, but increases in continuing program costs should not.

The second crucial consideration is the proper calculation of continuing costs. Perhaps the most critical part of this issue is accounting for the impact of inflation and increases in demand.[4] Exhibits 4-11 and 4-12 illustrate the importance of identifying the impact of these factors on a local government budget. What appear to be drastic spending increases in Town Appropriations are revealed in Exhibit 4-11 to actually be spending reductions once the impact of inflation is determined. Similarly, Exhibit 4-12 notes the rates of per capita spending for particular services. If we accept the use of town population as an adequate measure of service demand and correct for the impact of inflation, real spending has been cut considerably rather than having grown out of control! In most cases, the apparent dramatic increases are shown to be reductions in expenditures per person served.

Exhibit 4-12   Comparing Costs on Per Capita Basis

Budget Category	1971	1980	% Change
General Government	$ 8.89	$ 8.54	- 3.9%
Planning & Community Development	2.09	1.09	-47.5
Properties & Natural Resources	9.69	7.48	-22.8
Public Works	40.05	26.83	-32.9
Community Safety	46.12	44.69	- 3.0
Education	151.20	138.94	- 8.1
Hospital	-	7.96	-
Human Resources	10.65	7.47	-29.8
Library	7.84	6.10	-22.1

Thus, the use of graphs, tables, and text to document the true costs of service delivery is important to an agency. Exhibit 4-13 shows a simple method local governments can use to calculate the impact of inflation. **Agencies, budget officials, chief executives, and elected officials should be aware of the way such forces as inflation and service demands impact the budget, regardless of what final use they may make of such data.** Everyone in the budget process should try to communicate openly and honestly, while working toward their particular goals in the context of

Exhibit 4-13   Using Implicit Price Deflator

Calculating the impact of inflation is not a terribly difficult proposition. Essentially, you compare current prices to prices in a previous year, called the base year, to produce a price ratio. Current expenditures are then divided by the ratio to determine what you would be spending in the current year if there had been zero inflation. This figure is called constant dollar expenditures, meaning what you would have spent if the value of a dollar had been constant, rather than inflated.

The Implicit Price Deflator for State and Local Government Purchases of Goods and Services has been developed using price ratios for the items usually bought by these governments. It is published by the U.S. Government in the Survey of Current Business. To use the deflator to determine the impact of inflation on a current agency budget from any base year you should:

1. Divide the current IPD by 100.
2. Divide current spending by the quotient from #1.
3. Divide the base year IPD (choose any year to which you wish to compare current spending) by 100.
4. Multiply the quotient from #2 times the quotient from #3 to give constant dollar expenditures (what current purchases would cost if there had been zero inflation since the base year).

As an example, suppose you wish to determine the impact of inflation on your six-year-old agency since it was established. Assume first year spending was $70,000, current expenditures are $100,000, the current year IPD is 175, and the base year (six years ago) IPD was 125. Dividing 175 by 100 equals 1.75. Dividing $100,000 by 1.75 equals $57,142. Dividing 125 by 100 equals 1.25. Multiplying $57,142 by 1.25 equals $71,428. Virtually the entire increase in spending over six years is due to inflation, not real budget increases.

overall governmental needs. Presenting budget data in per capita and/or inflation-adjusted terms helps promote a more accurate and detailed understanding of agency expenditure plans and is not difficult or time consuming. Therefore, it is useful for local governments and agency directors to examine spending plans in such terms.

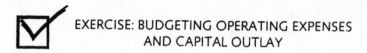

EXERCISE: BUDGETING OPERATING EXPENSES AND CAPITAL OUTLAY

1. You are the staff assistant to the Director of Agency X and among your responsibilities is preparation of the operating expense and capital outlay portions of the agency's annual budget request for the 1990-1991 fiscal year. One of your agency's programs provides an identification card to any citizen who seeks one. A portion of the budget history of this program is as follows:

CATEGORY	1987-88 ACTUAL	1988-89 ACTUAL	1989-90 ESTIMATE
Supplies	$1995	$2207	$2400
Utilities	$ 512	$ 985	$1500
Repairs	$ 0	$ 210	$1200
Training	$ 125	$ 125	$ 125
Travel	$ 577	$ 410	$ 100

Assume the following facts:

- In 1988-89, 1650 citizens were served.
- Projections are that in 1990-1991, 200 citizens will request services.
- The estimated price deflator for 1990-1991 is 110.0, using 1988-89 = 100.0 as the base year.
- The Chief Executive has stated that no new or improved programs will be included in this year's budget due to a lack of revenue.
- In addition, no new equipment requests will be approved.
- Although not a "glamour" agency, your program and performance are usually supported adequately by both the Chief Executive and the legislative body.
- The total budget for your local government is small enough that your agency is reviewed with care by the Budget Office.

The following "tools" and techniques are available to you:

- unit costs
- incremental analysis

64   PRACTICAL GOVERNMENT BUDGETING

- inflation adjustments
- political "savvy"
- knowledge of continuing, new, and improved programs
- trend-line projections

Using all of the above information, construct a budget request for supplies, utilities, repairs, training, and travel, including a narrative rationale. Be prepared to present the mathematics **and justification** behind your request in detail. Attach any supplemental materials you would like.

2. One of Agency Y's functions is to transport office furniture and equipment to the various buildings in which the local government staff is located. Your performance objective is to complete 100% of the moves on the date scheduled. This year you achieved 50% success on this objective. Your agency hopes to replace one vehicle and add one new vehicle for these purposes. The Budget Office sends you Exhibit 4-9 in response to your request for guidance on how to proceed.

Your current vehicles are a six-year-old Chevrolet S-10 truck with 91,000 miles (Property Control Number 783) and a two-year-old four door Ford Tempo with 7,000 miles (Property Control Number 941). The truck was out of service due to repairs for 46 workdays during the past six months. The Tempo has required nothing but gasoline.

Types of vehicles currently available for purchase under the government's vehicle purchase program are Chevrolet Cavalier midsize sedans at $9250, Chevrolet Celebrity Station Wagons at $10,900, and Chevrolet G-10 1/2 Ton Vans at $10,800.

Prepare the necessary budget requests for vehicles in this format:

ITEM	UNIT COST	NO. OF ITEMS	TOTAL COST	NEW OR REPLACEMENT

Please provide justification for all requests.

1. *Uniform Accounting System* (Tallahassee, Florida: State of Florida Department of Banking and Finance, June, 1988).

2. Edward A. Lehan, *Simplified Governmental Budgeting* (Chicago, Illinois: Municipal Finance Officers Association, 1981), p. 25.

3. Leo Herbert *et. al.*, *Governmental Accounting and Control* (Monterey, California: Brooks-Cole, 1984), p. 232.

4. This section, including Exhibits 4-11 and 4-12, is based upon "A Brief Look at Arlington's Budget," in Carol W. Lewis and A. Grayson Walker III, *Casebook in Public Budgeting and Financial Management* (Englewood Cliffs, New Jersey: Prentice-Hall, 1984), pp. 185-86.

Chapter 5

DEFENDING BUDGET PROPOSALS _____

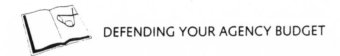

DEFENDING YOUR AGENCY BUDGET

HOW THIS CHAPTER WILL BE USEFUL

The preparation of an agency budget request is not an easy task. The head of the agency must produce a request that is not only compatible with the local government's fiscal and management policies but also fulfills the needs of the individual agency. The agency head must submit a reasonable and feasible budget request and also be able to **defend** that proposal.

The ideal situation in local government would be to have enough revenues to cover all agencies' original budget requests. Unfortunately, this is rarely the case. Usually, there is a constant balancing act to bring the estimated revenues and proposed expenditures into balance. This process can be rather lengthy and cumbersome since most agencies view the budget process from their perspective of "getting as much as we can." Unless an agency is part of an Enterprise or Internal Service Fund most agencies never consider the revenue side of the budget process when preparing their requests.

In light of this ongoing balance process, there is a real need for the agency head to sufficiently defend his budget request. This chapter will focus on two major areas in this "budget defense" process. First, we will discuss the agency head's role in preparing and justifying his budget needs. The agency head must be able to successfully "sell" his budget proposal to the various budget reviewers. Here we will focus on the written presentation of the budget as opposed to the technical preparation discussed in the two previous chapters. Second, we will look at reviewing an agency's budget submittal from three different perspectives: the Central Budget Office, the Chief Executive (City Manager, County Administrator), and the Legislature (elected officials such as City Council or County Commission).

Exhibit 5-1   Revenues Impose Limits

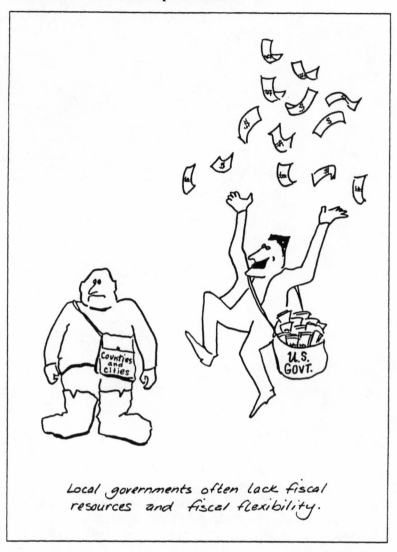

Local governments often lack fiscal resources and fiscal flexibility.

The purposes of this chapter are to enable you to:

1. Discuss the differences between mandatory, base, and discretionary expenditures.

2. Identify and discuss the three perspectives by which an agency budget is reviewed.

3. Prepare a written justification for a budget submittal.

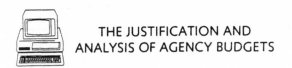

Strategies Versus Justification

The two previous chapters provided you with information on how to prepare a budget from the technical standpoint. This chapter will focus on the agency preparing a narrative defense for the dollars requested.

In real estate, the main selling point of a piece of property or a home is *location-location-location.* In budget proposals, the main selling point is *justification-justification-justification.* All too often agencies rely on various strategies and tactics when preparing their budget requests for the Central Budget Office, Chief Executive, and the Legislature rather than preparing solid justifications. The main objective of these games is for the agency to retain the base budget and, if at all possible, increase it over current-year appropriations.

In his book, *The Politics of the Budgetary Process,* Aaron Wildavsky identifies several of these agency strategies,[1] including:

- Cutting popular programs, knowing full well they will be restored.

- Asking for all or nothing on the grounds that the program will not be viable with further cuts.

- Merging new or challenged programs with popular programs so that they will be less susceptible to attack.

- Claiming new activities are really "old stuff" and part of the base.

- Maintaining appropriations at present level while using funds for other purposes.

- Starting new programs with small sums, knowing the opening wedge will be enlarged in later years.

- Claiming some expenditures are only temporary.

- Using workload data to build up the budget base.

- Arguing that a program, through user fees/charges, will pay for itself.

- Demonstrating that expenditure increases now will result in savings later.

- Capitalizing on a crisis to initiate new activities.

This list of strategies is by no means all inclusive! However, it is very real and it is tempting for agency heads to try such tactics at some point in time during their budget preparation career. When utilizing these strategies in the budget preparation/proposal process, agency heads feel that there is no need to have to fully justify their requests.

Sometimes these strategies work. However, more often these strategic games result in the reverse effect for the agency. After all, the Central Budget Office, the Chief Executive, and the Legislature are all cognizant of these ploys and often end up playing "hard ball" with the agency. The "all or nothing" strategy may result in an agency ending up with zero dollar ($0) allocations. Or, the

Exhibit 5-2   Spenders and Cutters

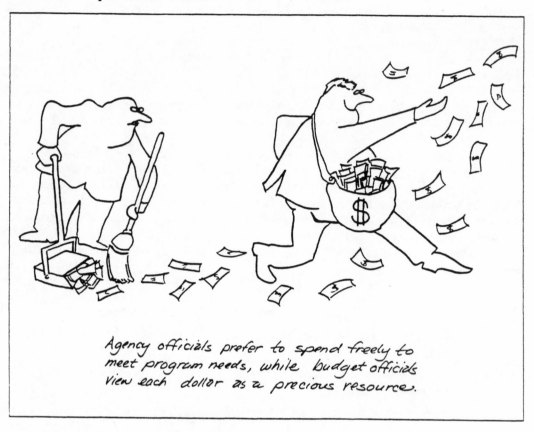

Agency officials prefer to spend freely to meet program needs, while budget officials view each dollar as a precious resource.

agency may have to provide the budget reviewers with an in-depth analysis as to how a user fee oriented program will actually pay for itself. Finally, the agency head runs the risk of losing credibility as a responsible manager if there is no substantial information to back up the funding requests.

Mandatory, Base, and Discretionary Expenditures

Instead of relying on budget games and strategies, it is usually better for the agency head to **justify** the need for his budget expenditure requests. Expenditures should be justified in three separate categories: mandatory, base, and discretionary.

Mandatory expenditures are those that are required by federal, state, or local law. Such expenditures include social security contributions, pension/retirement, unemployment compensation, bargaining unit agreement items, as well as general obligation debt payments. The payment of employees' salaries could be considered mandatory. However, there may be some "discretion" as to the number of employees an agency "really needs" to operate at its expected service level. Justification for these items normally consists of citing the federal, state, or local law or mandate that resulted in this cost being considered mandatory. Budget reviewers are usually aware of the mandatory costs of an agency and are not looking to cut these items.

70

In the second category, **base expenditures** relate to those items that are considered necessary and essential to the agency's continuing operations. This category would include the agency's major operating expenses such as rent, utilities, fuel, vehicle/equipment repair and maintenance, tools and implements, printing, general office supplies, and any other related items. The agency's justification for these expenses can come from reviewing actual prior year expenditure information, current budget year appropriations, as well as projecting the current year expenditures. Most agency heads are fully aware of the level of service that they are providing to the public. By looking at the prior year expenditure data, the agency head can determine how much it costs to provide this service. He should also be able to explain any major increases or decreases to the operating expenditures. For example, drastic increases in the Parks and Recreation budget request for operating expenses might be explained by the acquisition of new parks in the current fiscal year.

Even though some expenditure areas are considered as "base," an agency should always make sure that it retains workload data related to these areas. Availability of relevant and pertinent workload data could ease any pressure by the Legislature to "reduce or cut" those programs that are perceived as not performing at the desired service level. Also, in the event a local government decided to prepare budget proposals utilizing a Zero-Base Budget concept, the agency would have to be able to defend **all** expenses: mandatory, base, and discretionary. Lastly, evidence of productivity improvements is always welcomed by budget reviewers.

In the third category, **discretionary expenditures** are those items/activities that normally enhance the existing level of service. These expenditures are not essential to the success of the agency's operations, but often make the program function more effectively and efficiently or may enhance the public's perspective of the service level being provided. An example of discretionary expenditures might be the addition of 10 Deputies to the Sheriff's Department. The addition of the staff would hopefully decrease response time to emergency calls, increase the morale of the "overworked" Deputies, as well as heighten the public's feelings of "being safe" and putting their tax dollars to good use. The Sheriff's Department could, however, still function effectively with no new personnel.

In order to obtain funding for the additional personnel, the agency head will have to **justify** the need for this request. When discretionary expenditures are being requested, it is imperative that the agency "sell" the budget reviewers on their proposal with the written justification. **The justification for these discretionary expenditures should be written as if this is the only chance the agency will ever have to plead its case for the proposal.** In providing justification for new personnel requests, agencies should consider the following questions:

- Is there sufficient workload and performance data provided to support the request?
- Is the new position request the direct result of the implementation of a federal or state mandated program?
- Are there any local legal requirements that have resulted in the request for new personnel?
- Has the legislative body directed an increase in the service level that requires additional personnel?

Once the proposal has been written, the agency head/budget preparer should have an objective person read and comment on it. If this person is not sold on the idea, then a more effective presentation needs to be developed. Exhibit 5-3 provides a sample budget justification requesting new personnel.

Exhibit 5-3   Sample New Personnel Justification

```
Department/Division: Building Permits
Position Request:    Permits Clerk

Justification: This  division  currently  complies  with  the  Council's
commitment to issue a building permit within three days from the time it is
received in this office. Since last fiscal year, this office has experienced
over a 15% increase in the number of permits being requested (FY86-87, 2600
permits; FY87-88, 3000 permits). The staff size, however, has remained
constant over the past three years. In FY 87-88, over $10,000 of overtime
was paid to the existing Permit Clerks in order to comply with the three-
day issuance commitment. If the building rate continues as it has in prior
years, it is not only unreasonable, but also costly to continue working our
existing employees at this pace in order to keep up with the demands. Based
on the following calculations, this office could have hired one additional
Permits Clerk last year for the same cost paid in overtime to the four
existing clerks:

    Overtime: 4 clerks x 5 hours/week x $10.50 per hour
              x 52 weeks = $10,920/year (note - overtime is paid at time
              and a half. The Permits Clerk existing pay rate is $7/hour,
              overtime is $10.50/hour)

    Additional Clerk: 1 clerk x $6/hour x 35 hours/week
                      x 52 weeks = $10,920/year (note - $6/hour is starting pay for
                      the position)

In light of the above information, the Permits Office respectfully submits
its request for an additional Permits Clerk.
```

As stated earlier, workload or performance data is extremely useful in defending and supporting an agency's budget request. The agency must also consider the politically sensitive nature of the proposal as well. If the discretionary request is one that is related to the "health, welfare, and safety" of the citizens, then the agency should use this to its advantage. Obviously this can be construed as another ploy or strategy to convince the budget reviewers of the importance of the request. However, the budget reviewers are equally aware of such politically important programs.

Thus far this section has dealt specifically with the justification of an agency's proposed expenditures. However, there is another aspect that agencies need to bear in mind when preparing their budget requests—the revenue side of budgeting. If an agency is part of an Enterprise or Internal Service Fund, then it is more concerned with revenue estimates. However, for those agencies that are funded by general city/county/statewide revenues, the need for detailed justification is even more critical. Each agency may view its function as the most important to the local government, however, they are but an integral part of the **entire** operation. This realization does not diminish the role of each agency but should make it more aware of the "big picture" in terms of revenues, as well as expenditures.

Justification is the main ingredient to the success of an agency's budget proposal. The more workload/performance data available to support the request the better. The agency should also remember to write its budget proposal justification as if this is the only opportunity the agency will have to plead its case for the budget request.

72   PRACTICAL GOVERNMENT BUDGETING

Exhibit 5-4   Budget Reviews

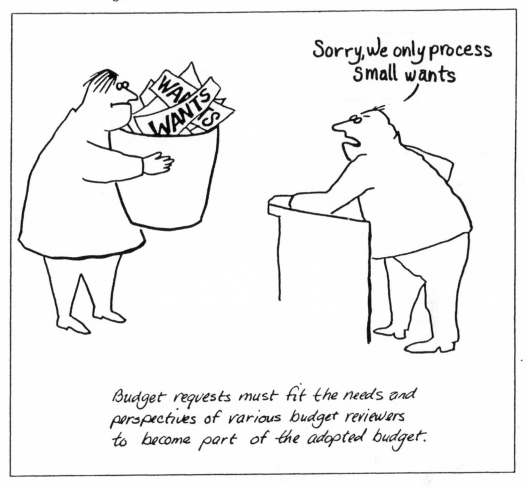

Three Perspectives of an Agency's Budget Review

This section of the chapter will identify and discuss three different points of view involved in the review of an agency's budget proposal. The perspectives involved are the Central Budget Office, Chief Executive, and the Legislature.

First, however, we need to identify the areas most likely to be the focus of the reviewer analyzing budget requests. Close attention is paid to expenditures that are:

- Discretionary rather than mandatory.
- Large, rather than small.
- Increasing, rather than decreasing or stable.

This means that **a proposal for a large, discretionary increase in appropriations will, in all likelihood, get plenty of analytical attention, while the small, recurring or mandatory items may not.**[2]

Budget reviewers also have to consider the availability of sufficient revenues when reviewing agency budget requests. This is an aspect of the budgeting process that most agencies are not concerned with. Revenue estimations are important because they drive the budget process. Agencies may ask for budget allocations which they feel are reasonable and feasible; however, if there are not sufficient revenues, the "reasonableness" of the request is a moot point.

In conjunction with revenue considerations, budget reviewers are cognizant of the **entire** local government structure and its needs. Each agency's function plays an integral part in the success of the organization. However, the ultimate task of the budget reviewers is to determine how estimated revenues can best be appropriated so that the organization operates in the most effective and efficient manner while providing an acceptable level of all services.

The Central Budget Office's Review

The role of the central budget office in the budget process is probably the most crucial and difficult. The budget office not only has to review budget requests keeping the agencies' needs in mind, but also has to consider the chief executive and legislative policies, programs and other preferences. In his book, *Budgeting For Modern Government*, Donald Axelrod describes how budget offices approach this delimma:[3]

> Central budget offices see themselves as bastions of objectivity, rising above the parochial concerns of agencies. They pride themselves on sensitivity to the needs of an entire country or state and not just to special segments of the public ... Only the budget office, in its view, ferrets out inefficiency and ineffectiveness in programs and makes sure that the public gets appropriate value for the money invested in the budget.

In attempting to make these "objective" agency recommendations, the central budget office is fully aware of:

- the fiscal and management policies of the organization
- the fiscal condition of the local government
- the political climate that influences budget recommendations

The fiscal and management policies are normally set forth by the Legislature as recommended by the Chief Executive. Such policies used as guidelines by the budget office could include the following:

- No tax increase
- No new personnel
- No new vehicles: only recommend replacement of existing vehicles as needed
- No expansion of programs
- No increase in levels of service

The items identified above give the budget office an idea as to how to review agency budget requests and what recommendations would be appropriate. For example, it would not be prudent for a Budget Analyst to spend a great deal of time analyzing the Planning and Zoning Department's requests for three new vehicles and three new planners when a directive regarding the vehicles and positions has already been issued.

The fiscal condition of the organization equates to the availability of revenues to support the agency requests. **Revenues drive the budget process.** Revenue estimates are normally done in conjunction with the budget review and recommendation process. These estimates may be provided by a Finance or Comptroller's Office, or the Central Budget Office itself may perform revenue projections. This simultaneous process is important because it allows the budget office staff to make recommendations on agency requests in light of the projected fiscal condition of the local government.

Awareness of the political climate of the organization is crucial to the budget office when reviewing agency budget requests. This is important to the budget office because "untimely attacks on popular programs—programs which are defined as basic or vital or programs regarded as 'sacred cows' by powerful interests—can produce negative returns for budget analysts."[4] By being aware of the political program preferences, the budget office can avoid needlessly analyzing programs that are a "given." This awareness can also save the budget office the dreaded task of explaining to the elected body that their most favored, but fiscally unreasonable, program was cut from the budget. On the other hand, this also provides the budget office with more time to review other discretionary expenditure requests.

While the agency head prepares and justifies the budget proposal in terms of mandatory, base, and discretionary expenditures, the budget office reviews budget requests in the same manner. Mandatory expenditures are uncontrollable and have to be funded. The budget office normally reviews these expenditure requests to insure that the agencies have *sufficient* allocations. For example, are there enough monies requested for employee salaries, Social Security contributions, pension payments, or bargaining unit agreement items? **Budget offices can and do recommend increases in budget requests when appropriate.**

Base expenditure requests are reviewed to insure that there are no major increases in these items, **unless** there is sufficient and appropriate justification. The budget office will make its recommendations based on prior year actual information, current budget year allocations, as well as projected expenditures for the current year.

Discretionary expenditure requests are scrutinized more closely than mandatory or base expenditure requests. A strong justification is required in such instances based upon detailed documentation or new policy initiatives supported by elected officials. The budget office may approve a few of these items, resources permitting. However, since these types of expenditures are not required for the agency to function adequately, then the budget office will more than likely not recommend the expenditure. If the agency feels strongly about the expenditure, then the agency head can normally appeal to the chief executive or the legislature. However, the agency head must be cautious about utilizing such an appeal process! If the expenditure request was denied because it was considered as one of the "no" items on the fiscal and management policies list, the agency head runs the very real risk of losing the battle, as well as falling into "disfavor" with the chief executive and/or legislature.

As stated earlier, the central budget office has a difficult task in the budget review process. While trying to make reasonable budget recommendations for individual agencies, the budget office must also keep in mind the fiscal and management policies of the Legislature. However, if an agency does manage to get their requests approved by the budget office, it stands a good chance of winning the approval of the chief executive and the legislature.

The Chief Executive's Review

The role of the chief executive during the budget review process is to carry out the policies and directives of the legislative body. This is usually accomplished by the chief executive working closely with the central budget office to insure that the policies and directives are followed during its review of agency budget requests.

Once the budget office has completed its review of all agency requests, it makes its recommendations to the chief executive. The majority of the time, these recommendations will be supported by the chief executive who then passes the same recommendations to the legislature for their approval. However, there are additional considerations the chief executive must focus on during his budget review stage.

First, the chief executive must feel comfortable that the recommendations of the budget office are appropriate and have taken into account all the fiscal and management policies/directives outlined earlier in the budget review process. This step serves as a check to make sure the policies are being adhered to.

Second, the chief executive must determine that there are no excessively controversial items recommended in the budget to the legislature. For instance, he certainly does not want to recommend a new program in the budget that the legislature had previously disapproved in the current budget year. Sometimes an agency will try this tactic, but it is usually not very successful, nor is it wise!

Third, the chief executive must review the budgets to make sure that those "politically preferred programs" are included in the recommendations. Frequently, these may be programs that are not fiscally reasonable, but are politically powerful. The placement of the same number of school crossing guards at **each** elementary school in a county or district is not a financially reasonable decision. Some schools might have less traffic than others or fewer students to "cross." However, this is an area that deals with the health, safety, and welfare of young children. Therefore, no matter how fiscally wrong a decision might be, the chief executive must consider the political ramifications if such a recommendation is not made. The main concern here, after the welfare of the children, is to protect the legislature and the executive from any "potentially explosive situations."

The Legislature's Review

The legislature's review and ultimate recommendations on the budget depends on: (1) the quality of the chief executive's review and resulting recommendations and (2) the way in which these recommendations are submitted to the legislature:

> Legislative review of the budget depends first and foremost on the way in which budget programs are presented by the executive . . . A budget presentation which is overdetailed and is not supported by clearly descriptive narratives produces legislative ineptitude, frustration, and resentment. Clarity in budget presentation carries over to clarity in appropriation structure.[5]

As the comments above indicate, the legislature wants and needs budget information from the executive which can be easily read and understood. Few local government legislative bodies have the kind of staff assistance necessary to research budget issues independently. Thus, clarity and brevity of the budget information for review are essential. If the chief executive has performed his role properly in the budget review/recommendation process, then the legislature should have a budget with which it feels comfortable.

However, even if the chief executive has done a good job in his review/recommendation role, the legislature will often feel that it cannot simply "rubberstamp" the budget recommendations. They "owe it to the taxpayers" to be certain that there are no frivolous expenditures in the budget. In such

PRACTICAL GOVERNMENT BUDGETING

cases, the legislative body will search out and make some cuts that the legislators feel are warranted. Reductions will usually be made in discretionary expenditures.

On the other hand, the legislature will also review the budget to make sure that individual legislator's "pet projects" are included in the budget. These may consist of projects that legislators have promised their district residents would be included in the budget recommendations, such as particular road improvements or monies for more police protection in a high crime area. If these items have **not** been included in the chief executive's recommendations, then the legislature would have to get majority approval to add them to the budget.

Finally, the legislature wants a "controversy-free" budget. If there are any questionable items in the budget, then the legislature needs to know. The members do not want to be caught off guard, particularly since they are charged with the ultimate approval of the budget.

The budget preparation/review/recommendation process is very lengthy and involved. While the public may see only the finished product (that is, the legislature's approved budget), the final budget is actually the result of an elaborate, lengthy, and incremental budget review process.

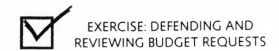 EXERCISE: DEFENDING AND REVIEWING BUDGET REQUESTS

1. As Public Safety Director (the Sheriff) of Ocean County, you are requesting the creation of an additional patrol zone during the budget process. The zone would require four new Deputy positions at an annual cost of $250,000. (This figure includes all costs—personnel, operating, and capital). Now that you have calculated how much it would cost to fund these positions, your task is to prepare the written justification for the positions.

All agency heads have been advised by the County Administrator that there should be no requests for new personnel and that the County Council has indicated that they want **no property tax increase next year**. Since the Public Safety operations are funded by countywide ad valorem taxes, this makes the task of getting the new positions approved even more difficult.   ↳ pROpeRty

In preparing your budget request, you have gathered basic statistical data regarding Public Safety's activities in the requested zone, as well as countywide. The information collected is as follows:

Countywide

- Average number of calls per zone is 450 per month
- 55% of the calls are "nuisance calls"—complaints of noisy dogs, teenagers, etc.—while 45% of the calls are "serious crime calls"—rape, robberies, murders, etc.
- Response time for emergency calls countywide is 10 minutes
- Response time for nonemergency calls is 13 minutes
- The countywide population has increased 15% over last year

Requested Zone

- Average number of calls is 560 per month, 45% of which are "nuisance calls" and 55% are "serious crime calls"
- Response time for emergency calls is 15 minutes

- Response time for nonemergency calls is 25 minutes

- The population in the requested zone has increased 25% over last year due to the opening of a new subdivision

Based on the information above, prepare your written justification for the creation of an additional patrol zone that would require hiring four new Deputies.

2. You are a Budget Analyst for the Ocean County Central Budget Office. Review the request above, as well as the statistical data given. As a budget reviewer, consider and respond to the following questions:

- What are the fiscal and management policies that must be considered in reviewing and making a recommendation on this request?

- What might be the impact upon the requested zone's activities if the additional positions are not approved?

- Do you feel that there is sufficient data provided by the Public Safety Director to present a good justification? If no, what additional data would be helpful?

NOTES

1. Aaron Wildavsky, *The Politics of the Budgetary Process*, 3rd edition (Boston, Massachusetts: Little, Brown and Company, 1979), pp. 63-126.

2. Edward A. Lehan, *Simplified Governmental Budgeting*, (Chicago, Illinois: Municipal Finance Officers Association, 1981), p. 63.

3. Donald Axelrod, *Budgeting for Modern Government* (New York, New York: St. Martins Press, 1988), p. 71.

4. Lehan, *op. cit.*, p. 63.

5. Jesse Burkhead, *Government Budgeting* (New York, New York: John Wiley and Sons, 1956), p. 311.

_____

Chapter 6

PREPARING REVENUE ESTIMATES _____

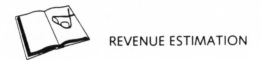 REVENUE ESTIMATION

HOW THIS CHAPTER WILL BE USEFUL

The previous chapters in this _Workbook_ have all focused on the expenditure side of budget preparation. This chapter will discuss how revenue estimates are prepared and the importance of this activity in the budget preparation process.

During the budget preparation process, most agency heads are primarily concerned with developing a reasonable budget request. Efforts are made to at least get the same monetary allocations as in the current budget year, while also trying to get "a little bit more" for the next year. Unless the agency is funded in an Enterprise or Internal Service Fund, most agency heads are not involved in the revenue side of the budget process.

Nevertheless, it is important that agency heads and public managers become familiar with the revenue estimating function of the budget process. As stated before, revenues drive the budget process. If there are not sufficient revenues available to allocate to the agencies, then the reasonableness or the urgency of their requests is a moot point. Moreover, the growing emphasis on "pay-as-you-go" approaches and user fees is involving more managers in the revenue side of budgeting.

Revenue estimation is more an art than a science. It depends upon future events, and most of them involve uncontrollable factors such as changing economic conditions and population growth or decline. Therefore, any major changes in the economy or population growth can have a detrimental effect on revenue collections.

There is no "tried and true" formula for projecting revenues. The majority of local government revenue proejections are based on historical collection trends, as well as the fiscal posture and climate of the current budget year. In addition, there are certain criteria that revenue estimators consider when making their projections. This chapter will include the following two major sections in order to discuss these factors:

‚ Description of Funds and Major Revenue Categories
• The Revenue Estimatation Process

It is intended that the information contained in this chapter will help you understand more about the revelance and importance of this function of the budget process.

OBJECTIVES

Upon concluding this chapter, you should be able to:

1. Identify the seven major revenue categories utilized by local governments in revenue projections.

2. Identify and describe five revenue estimating models.

3. Explain why the simplistic model of revenue estimation is the most commonly used by local governments.

4. Prepare reasonable revenue estimates based on historical data made available to you.

ESTIMATING REVENUES
BY FUNDS AND CATEGORIES

Description of Funds and Major Revenue Categories

Prior to actually estimating revenues, one must be familiar with the fund structure of the local government. This includes not only the **classification of funds** that the local government utilizes, but also the **major categories of revenues** available to the jurisdiction. The description of funds and major revenue categories varies across the states, but the information that follows in this section should be applicable to most local governments.[1]

Classification of Funds

The source of funding for an agency's budget can determine the types of recommendations made for the next budget year. If an agency is funded by general city-, county-, or statewide revenues, then the budget requests are scrutinized more closely than if an agency generates its own income as part of an Enterprise or Internal Service Fund. So that you, as budget preparers, can understand the differences in this "scrutinizing" process, it is important to understand the various classification of funds which a local government is required to use.

As defined by the Generally Accepted Accounting Principles (GAAP), a fund is a set of interrelated accounts which record assets (revenues) and liabilities (expenditures/obligations) related to a specific purpose. These are fairly standard from place to place. For example, one widely-used system includes seven fund groups, as identified below (the detailed description of these fund groups can be found in Chapter 1).

- 001 General Fund
- 100 Special Revenue Funds
- 200 Debt Service Funds
- 300 Capital Project Funds
- 400 Enterprise Funds
- 500 Internal Service Funds
- 600 Trust and Agency Funds

One should note that there are numerical codes associated with each fund group. These numerical codes are unique to the group. For instance, all Debt Service Funds will be part of a "200" series fund grouping—Fund 201 could be Library Debt Service, Fund 202 could be Correctional Facility Debt Service, and so on. This numerical designation makes it very easy for one to recognize the fund type.

Generally speaking, there is a minimal amount of agency input in projecting revenues for the General, Special Revenue, Debt Service, and Capital Project Funds. Normally, the office or individuals charged with the revenue estimating responsibility makes these projections. Agencies *are* involved in this process if they are part of an Enterprise or Internal Service Fund. This is expected since the agency head should be familiar with its *entire* operation. For instance, the Solid Waste Agency Head should know enough about his enterprise fund operation to assist in projecting revenue receipts. If the agency head does not know enough about his operations to make recommendations on the revenue side of his budget, then the organization has some serious problems!

Major Categories of Revenue

All local governments categorize their major sources of revenue. This is done so that one can easily determine where the revenues are coming from to support the organization's operations. The seven categories of revenues most commonly used by local governments are as follows:

- Taxes
- Licenses and Permits
- Intergovernmental Revenues
- Charges for Services
- Fines and Forfeitures
- Miscellaneous Revenues
- Non-Revenues

Taxes are charges levied by a local unit against the income or wealth of a person or corporation. The ad valorem tax, or the property tax, is usually a local government's largest single revenue source. (Chapter 7 will be dedicated entirely to estimating property taxes.) Additional forms of taxes levied are sales and use taxes such as a Tourist Development Tax, Gas Tax, or Utility Tax.

Licenses and Permits include revenues derived from the issuance of local licenses and permits such as occupational licenses, building permits, motor vehicles licenses, or well permit fees.

Intergovernmental Revenues account for all revenues received from federal, state, or other local government sources in such forms as grants or shared revenues. Examples of this revenue type are State Library Construction Grants, Criminal Justice Grants, or State Revenue-Sharing dollars.

Charges for Services reflect the receipt of revenues stemming from such sources as zoning fees, impact fees, legal aid fees, clerk's fees for copying/searching court records, water and sewer charges, or beach access fees.

Exhibit 6-1   General Fund Revenues by Major Category

Revenue Source	Actual 1986-87	Adopted 1987-88	Revised 1987-88	Budget 1988-89
General Fund				
TAXES				
Ad Valorem	$27,764,580	36,767,537	37,034,100	39,944,108
Ad Valorem Delinquent	158,091	75,000	125,000	125,000
Utility	0	0	0	2,000,000
TOTAL	27,922,671	36,842,537	37,159,100	42,069,108
LICENSES & PERMITS				
Occupational	90,000	100,000	70,000	75,000
INTERGOVERNMENTAL				
State Reimbursement	425,000	450,000	450,000	470,000
State Revenue Sharing	3,800,000	4,200,000	4,500,000	4,800,000
Beverage Licenses	160,000	165,000	165,000	168,000
TOTAL	4,385,000	4,815,000	5,115,000	5,438,000
CHARGES FOR SERVICES				
Sales of Maps, Books	14,478	12,000	15,000	15,000
County Officer Fees	1,183,055	1,000,000	1,000,000	1,100,000
Beach Access Fees	3,200,000	3,300,000	3,300,000	3,500,000
TOTAL	4,397,533	4,312,000	4,315,000	4,615,000
FINES & FORFEITURES				
Court Fines	880,000	725,000	800,000	850,000
MISCELLANEOUS				
Interest Income	891,782	600,000	700,000	650,000
Sale of Surplus Equip	105,000	25,000	40,000	250,000
Miscellaneous	19,180	23,500	23,500	24,000
TOTAL	1,015,962	648,500	763,500	924,000
NON-REVENUES				
Trust Fund Transfer	4,465,404	3,448,415	3,333,415	3,500,000
Loan Proceeds	0	700,000	700,000	1,500,000
Fund Balance	1,500,000	1,900,000	1,900,000	2,200,000
TOTAL	5,965,404	6,248,415	6,133,415	7,200,000
GENERAL FUND TOTAL	$ 44,656,570	53,691,452	54,356,015	61,171,108

Fines and Forfeitures include revenues received from fines and penalties imposed for the commission of statutory offenses, violations, and for neglect of official duty. Library fines and any fines paid through the courts are included in this revenue category.

Miscellaneous Revenue includes all revenue not classified in any of the above revenue categories. Interest income is the major revenue source in this category. Receipts from the sale of surplus equipment or rental of public property are also examples of miscellaneous revenue.

Non-Revenues are monies received by the government that are not new additions to assets of the government as a whole. These revenues include inter-fund transfers, bond/loan proceeds, and appropriated fund balances.

Exhibit 6-2   Revenue Projection Form

Fund: Municipal Service District (120)

Revenue Source: 1410

Revenue Title: Utility Tax

I. Revenues

---

(1) Actual Revenue 1986-87	(2) Current Budget 1987-88	(3) Revised Estimate 1987-88	(4) Revenue Estimate 1988-89
$6,500,000	$6,700,000	$6,700,000	$6,900,000

II. Revenue Explanations. Identify major variances between Budgeted Revenue, Revised Estimate, and Revenue Estimate (if any):

Dollar volume dependent on weather for remainder of 1987-88. Estimated increase for 1988-89 based on continuing population growth.

III. Revenue Description. Provide general information about the revenue source such as: are funds collected per state statute, ordinance, or resolution and can funds be used only for specific purposes?

Tax collected on all utilities (electricity, bottled gas etc.) for homes in the unincorporated area of the County. Funds are elected as per County Ordinance 85-121, adopted 4/15/85, effective 10/1/85. Revenue restricted to County Municipal Service District purposes only.

Contact Person:_____   Telephone:_____

Exhibit 6-1 details a local government's General Fund revenues by major category. Note that Taxes are in fact the major revenue source for the fund. This is common among local governments. Intergovernmental Revenues and Non-Revenues tend to be major sources of revenue as well since they include revenues such as State Revenue Sharing, Federal and State Grant monies, bond proceeds, inter-fund transfers, and appropriated fund balances.

Since these are the "big" revenue generating items, those persons performing the revenue estimating task will spend the majority of their time insuring that these revenue projections are as accurate as possible. There is not as much "margin of error" in large revenue sources as there is in the smaller revenue generating areas.

Now that we have discussed the major classification of funds and revenue categories, the next section of the chapter will focus on the actual Revenue Estimating Process.

Revenue Estimating Considerations

As stated earlier, revenue estimation is more an art than a science. However, the key to making good revenue projections includes the following general considerations:[2]

- A good understanding of the local government's revenue system.
- Understanding the factors that have affected past revenue collections.
- Having adequate and timely information with which to make projections.
- Exercising good judgement.

In most local governments, the task of estimating revenues is performed either by a Revenue or Comptroller's Office or the Central Budget Office. Usually there are only one or two people responsible for performing revenue estimates and these people become the local government's "experts" in revenue estimation. However, those agencies that are funded in an Enterprise or Internal Service Fund or which have an operation that generates substantial revenues that help in "covering the costs of operating" are often consulted in the revenue projecting process.

Exhibit 6-2 is an example of a Revenue Projection form that the "revenue projectors" might send to those agencies that have revenues associated with their operations. The "prior year" collections section would already be completed, however, the remainder of the information requested would be provided by the agency. This gives the agency an opportunity to make its own revenue projections. It also provides additional information for the revenue estimators to utilize in making their projections.

Revenue Estimation Models

In local government, there are five models that can be utilized when performing the revenue estimation task. They are as follows:

- **Simplistic Model**   This is revenue forecasting based on trend extrapolation of historical data, as well as taking into account changes in service demands that might affect revenue collections. Good judgement utilized in interpreting these trends is also a major factor used in this model.

- **Multiple Regression Model**   This is the utilization of independent variables, such as population and economy, to predict revenues.

- **Econometric Model**   This model bases revenue estimates on the simultaneous review of interdependent variables, such as the Consumer Price Index, interest rates, and construction activity.

- **Microsimulation Model**   Revenue estimates are made by using sample files of data, such as IRS returns, to predict future trends.

- **Input-Output Model**   This model uses sales and purchase data to determine where revenue is being generated.

The model most commonly used by local governments in making revenue projections is the **simplistic model**. This model is most useful to local governments in that it:

- is straightforward and uncomplicated
- requires data and financial records that are easily obtainable and accessible
- allows calculation of revenue projections rather simply and manually

Exhibit 6-3   The Art of Revenue Estimation

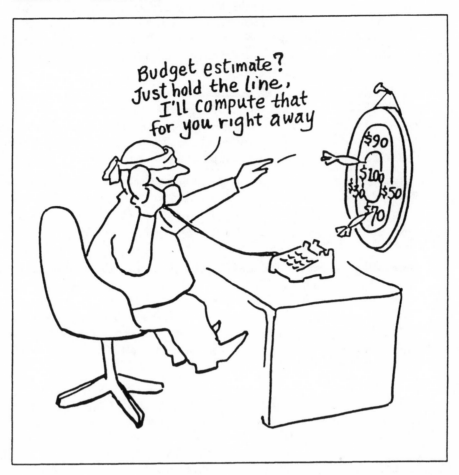

The next portion of this chapter will focus on procedures for estimating revenues. When discussing these procedures, we will be doing so in terms of utilizing the simplistic model of revenue estimation.

Procedures for Estimating Revenues

Every local government has a budget preparation / review / approval process that works for them. This is usually based on the organizational structure, legal/statutory requirements, and the preferences of the Chief Executive and Legislature. The procedures involved in estimating revenues are generally comparable in all local governments. The procedures detailed below are by no means all inclusive, however, they will give you a good idea as to the steps involved in the revenue estimating process:

> • **Project each revenue source separately.** This step is important because each revenue source is unique and distinct in its own right. "Taxes" as a general revenue source cannot

be estimated by itself since there are numerous forms of taxes. For example you might have property tax, gas tax, and utility tax in one fund, yet these are all taxes on different items. Therefore, it would not be prudent to try and estimate "Taxes" as one revenue source. In addition, making lots of small estimates instead of a few large ones reduces the impact of errors. In fact, over-estimates and under-estimates may even cancel each other out.

- **Concentrate on the revenue sources that generate the most revenue within a particular fund.** In a local government's General Fund, the property tax is usually the largest single source of revenue. Therefore, it is important that this figure is as accurate as possible. Usually it does not pay to spend a great deal of time on minor revenue sources that will not have a substantial impact on the fund.

- **Rely upon historical data in order to establish a trend in revenue collections.** The historical data that is available in an organization's financial records is probably the most critical source of information in making revenue projections. This information provides actual collections during previous fiscal years and is the basis for how trends in revenue collections are determined.

- **Account for seasonal or irregular fluctuations in past collections of each revenue source.** Special attention should be paid to this item. In a particular fiscal year, a local government may receive a one-time grant for a specific purpose. The revenue estimators need to take this into consideration so as not to "double up" or "over estimate" revenues for the upcoming fiscal year. This is the step in the revenue projection process where the experience of a long-time revenue estimator is important. One that is "new" to the process may not be familiar enough with this aspect to recognize that it is an "irregularity."

- **Project each revenue source in a conservative manner.** It is very important in the revenue projection process to underestimate your revenue projection rather than to overestimate them. The main reason for this is that once revenues are estimated and appropriated for expenditure, it is **extremely difficult** to go back to the Chief Executive and Legislature and tell them that there will, in fact, **not** be enough revenues to cover the estimated expenditures. This procedure for making revenue projections is nearly universal in local governments. Of course, revenue projections must still be as accurate as possible.

- **Use good judgement.** Often times local revenue estimators may be given revenue estimates from the State or even an agency head regarding a specific revenue source. If the historical trends reveal that this figure is completely out of line, then it is up to the person(s) performing the task of projecting revenues to use their best judgement in estimating a realistic figure. After all, they are ultimately responsible for all of the revenue projections for the local government.

Conclusion

Revenue estimation is a difficult art rather than a task which can be accomplished by a "tried and true" scientific method. Charles D. Liner has described the real revenue estimation process very well:[3]

The reader may be disappointed to find that no mathematical, statistical, or mechanical methods have been presented that would enable him to produce precise projections for each revenue source. Unfortunately, such techniques do not exist. We cannot produce adequate projections by feeding data into a computer. Rather, good projections must rest on thorough analysis, good judgement, realistic assumptions, and a sound approach.

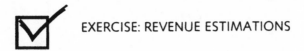 EXERCISE: REVENUE ESTIMATIONS

1. You are the person charged with the task of projecting revenues for Ocean County for Fiscal Year 1989. Exhibit 6-4 provides you with two years of prior year actual data as well as the adopted and estimated revenue figures for the current year. Please also consider the following factors:

Exhibit 6-4   Sample Revenue Estimation Data

Revenue Source	1986 Actuals	1987 Actuals	1988 Adopted	1988 Estimate	1989 Budget
Taxes					
Property	1659	1718	2202	2202	
Delinquent	12	13	8	8	
Franchise Fee	137	173	125	125	
Utility	6510	6677	7500	6900	
Licenses and Permits					
Occupational	213	220	220	220	
Contractors	19	19	18	18	
Building Permits	1265	1379	1350	1350	
Utility Use Fee	166	283	300	300	
Exam Fees	10	7	7	7	
Animal Licenses	13	19	17	21	
Sign Permits	40	28	20	30	
Well Permits	12	23	25	25	
Intergovernmental Revenues					
State Rev Sharing	156	173	165	170	
Charges for Services					
Zoning Fees	66	118	155	155	
Map Sales	36	80	85	85	
Planning Fees	31	93	70	110	
Storm Water Mgt	36	49	74	74	
Tree Preservation	7	7	7	7	

All figures expressed as thousands of dollars. Example, revenue from tree preservation program charges are $7,000 annually.

- The taxable value of property, the basis for estimating the property tax, is projected to increase by 8%.

- The Utility Tax is a tax levied on all utility use, primarily electricity. Due to an unusually warm winter in Ocean County, the "current estimate" for Utility Tax collections has been reduced by $600,000 over the earlier "current adopted" estimate made as part of the annual budget process for Fiscal Year 1988.

- Revenue sources associated with building/construction activity are anticipated to increase slightly, possibly 2-3%.

- All other revenue sources should follow historical trends in collections.

Review and analyze this data and then, based on the knowledge you have gained in this chapter regarding the estimation of revenues, complete the "Budget Request" column of Exhibit 6-4. This column represents the estimated revenue collections for each revenue source in the next fiscal year.

2. What revenue items account for the major sources of revenue for the Ocean County General Fund? Why do you think these are the major sources of revenue?

3. Identify those items that have major collection fluctuations. What might be the cause of these variances?

NOTES

1. The system presented here is used throughout the state of Florida. *Uniform Accounting System* (Tallahasee, Florida: State of Florida Department of Banking and Finance, June, 1988).

2. Charles D. Liner, "Projecting Local Government Revenue," in Jack Rabin *et. al., A Reader in Local Government Budgeting* (Athens, Georgia: Vinson Institute of Government, 1983), p. 83.

3. *Ibid.*, p. 91.

Chapter 7

UNDERSTANDING THE PROPERTY TAX

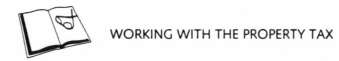

WORKING WITH THE PROPERTY TAX

HOW THIS CHAPTER WILL BE USEFUL

Most chapters in this *Workbook* familiarize local government line and staff public managers with the fundamentals of public budgeting as they are likely to experience it in directing their agencies. Therefore, a chapter on the property tax may seem a bit out of place. After all, it is elected officials who determine the property tax rate, and finance specialists like appraisers and tax collectors who administer it.

In addition, it is difficult to discuss the property tax without delving into the specifics of state systems, and there are as many systems as there are states! The specific types of property to be taxed, the ways in which these items are valued, the allowances for exemptions, and the procedures and limitations on how the tax may be applied are determined by state constitutions and legislation.

Nevertheless, the property tax remains the largest revenue source for most local governments in America, and the ability to set the property tax rate is perhaps the single most scrutinized action taken by a city, county, or school district in most years. **Therefore, we feel it is crucial for public managers to have a thorough understanding of the property tax process and to be able to relate their own agency budget to the property tax.** Since it is most effective to use concrete examples, we will describe the property tax system in the State of Florida as an illustration, but we will be emphasizing the essential elements of property taxes which apply everywhere. Still, readers should be sure to adjust the terms and concepts discussed here to the particular laws and regulations at work in their own state system.

Exhibit 7-1   Tax Revolts

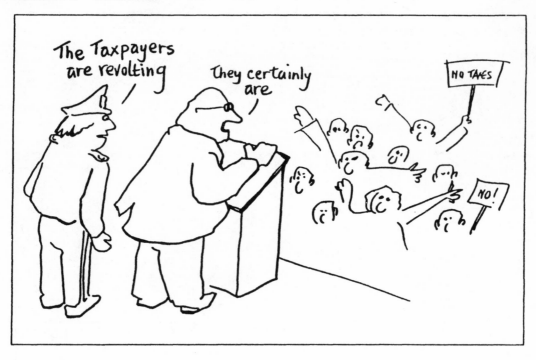

OBJECTIVES

This chapter should enable you to:

1. Describe the steps in determining the property tax rate from assessment to levy.

2. Analyze the budgetary implications of the various elements of property tax calculations including assessments, exemptions, tax base, tax levy, tax rate, and collections.

3. Explain the relationship between agency budgets and the property tax rate.

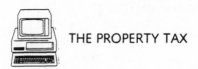   THE PROPERTY TAX

The property tax is highly unpopular with most citizens but it is a critical source of revenue for most local governments. It represents a large amount of money and is billed (though not necessarily paid) in a lump sum once a year, thereby magnifying its impact on taxpayers. It is not directly tied to any particular government services (as in the case of a user fee), thus leading to the complaint, "what am I getting for my taxes?" It is based on the inexact art of property assessment, leading to complaints about inequities and inconsistencies, some of which are possibly justified. It is generally collected by tax collectors on behalf of several jurisdictions, an administrative efficiency which nonetheless leads

Exhibit 7-2   Terms and Concepts for Determining the Tax Base

o **Assessed value** - A value established by the County Property Appraiser for all real or personal property for use as a basis for levying property taxes.

o **Exemption** - Amount deducted from the assessed value of property for tax purposes. Tax rates are applied to the balance, which is called the taxable value. Example: A 1980 amendment to the Florida Constitution sets the exemption for homesteads at $25,000. That means that a homeowner with property assessed at $50,000 would have to pay taxes on $25,000 of the assessment.

o **Property Appraiser** - The elected county official responsible for setting property valuations for tax purposes and for preparing the tax roll.

o **Property tax** - An ad valorem (according to value) tax paid on the fair market value of real property (land and buildings) and personal property

o **Real property** - Land and the buildings and other structures attached to it that are taxable under state law.

o **Tax base** - Total property valuations on which each taxing authority levies its tax rates.

o **Tax roll** - The master list of the assessed value of all taxable property within a government's jurisdiction. The list is prepared and certified by the Property Appraiser and presented to the various local governments which have property taxing authority each year.

o **Taxable value** - Assessed value of property minus exemptions.

to taxpayer confusion over just which local government or goverments are responsible for rate changes.

Considering all these facts, it is easy to understand why property tax revolt occurs. Government managers must respond to these problems by sharing the responsibilty of communicating to taxpayers the kinds and costs of services their agencies fund through this ad valorem tax.

In order to better understand the property tax process, it is necessary to follow it step by step. However, prior to "walking through" the process, one should be familiar with the terms and concepts in Exhibit 7-2. Then, we will use a local government in Florida during the mid-1980s as an example (see Exhibit 7-3). While specifics vary from state to state, every system must include the four steps of assessment, exemption, calculation, and collection discussed in this chapter. Finally, we will examine the property tax from the perspectives of the elected officials, the taxpaying citizen, and the government agency manager.

Step One—Assessment

The process begins with the determination of the amount of property subject to taxation. This is the job of the property tax appraiser, who must determine and certify the tax roll. This task is accomplished by listing all the items of taxable property in the county including land, homes, businesses, and equipment, determining the value of each, and deducting any exemptions from that value.

Exhibit 7-3   Sample Local Government Property Tax Profile

```
This data is used in Exhibit 7-5, 7-6, and 7-7 calculations.

Prior Year Millage                                    3.9314

Prior Year Taxable Values              $18,379,211,772

Prior Year Levy                            $72,256,033

Current Year Adjusted Value            $20,153,255,177

Current Year Taxable Value             $21,456,483,992

Rollback Proceeds                          $76,927,932

Rollback Rate                                         3.5853

Proposed Rate (Method 1)                              4.1300

Proposed Levy (Method 1)                   $88,570,107

Proposed Rate (Method 2)                              4.0000

Proposed Levy (Method 2)                   $85,825,932
```

According to state law in Florida, property must be assessed at "just" value, but that is more an art than a science. The statue defines just value to include such factors as cash value, use, locale, size, replacement cost, condition, income, and net sale proceeds. For the most part, the County Appraiser's staff and computer software attempt to identify comparable properties that have been sold recently to assign value. Every piece of property is reassessed each year, and appraisers on the county's staff in our example are responsible for about 5000 appraisals annually, or about 20 each working day.

Generally, the elected Appraiser is conservative, and few property owners would sell their property for the value assigned for tax purposes. The State of Florida does oversee the work of County Appraisers, however, doing its own research based on comparables. This prevents the county appraisers from being too generous in their estimates. Nonetheless, few property owners appeal their assessments. In our sample county, between 150 and 500 of over 250,000 parcels are appealed each year, less than 0.2 percent of the cases. An estimated 25% of them win reductions from the appraiser's office or from the Property Appraisal Adjustment Board, which consists of five elected officials. Although specifics vary, local property tax appraisal with some state supervision in the name of uniformity is typical across the nation.

Step Two—Exemptions and Other Reductions

Once assessed value has been determined, exemptions must be subtracted in order that taxable value can be determined. Property owned by governments or charitable, religious, and educational institutions is totally immune from taxation. There are also exemptions granted by the state legislature

Exhibit 7-4   Terms and Concepts for Property Tax Rates

o   **Levy** - The total value of property taxes authorized by a unit of government.

o   **Mill or millage** - 1/1000 (.001) of one dollar; property tax rate is usually expressed as millage rate of tax dollars per thousand dollars of taxable property value; determined by dividing total tax levy by total nonexempt assessed valuation and then multiplying by 1000. Thus, a city seeking to levy $1,000,000 in property taxes on property valued at $200,000,000 would be establishing a millage rate of $5 per thousand ($1 million divided by $200 million multiplied by 1000).

o   **Rolled back/rollback rate** - Defined by Florida TRIM law as the millage rate which, when multiplied times the tax base, exclusive of new construction added to that tax roll, would yield the same amount of revenue for the taxing authority as was yielded by the millage rate levied in the previous year. In normal circumstances, as the tax base rises by virtue of reassessment, the rolled back rate will be slightly lower than the previous year's millage rate.

o   **Truth in Millage Law (TRIM)** - A 1980 Florida law which changed the budget process for local taxing governments. It was designed to keep the public informed about the taxing intentions of the various taxing authorities.

Exhibit 7-5   Calculating the Property Tax: Method 1

o   STEP 1 - Determine total revenues required to operate government in the coming fiscal year.
     Example: $271,363,745

o   STEP 2 - Estimate anticipated revenues from all nonproperty tax sources.
     Example: $187,222,143

o   STEP 3 - Subtract Step 2 total from Step 1 total to determine amount of revenue which must be collected from property tax to balance the budget.
     Example: $ 84,141,602

o   STEP 4 - Divide Step 3 total by .95 in order to compensate for anticipated 5% uncollected taxes. The result is the tax levy.
     Example: $ 88,570,107

o   STEP 5 - Divide the levy by the tax base to determine the millage rate. Multiply the result by 1000 to express the tax rate in terms of tax dollars owed per thousand dollars of taxable property value.
     Example: $4.13 per thousand

UNDERSTANDING THE PROPERTY TAX

Exhibit 7-6   Calculating the Property Tax: Method 2

```
o      STEP 1 - Determine the tax rate which local officials plan to adopt.
       Example: $4.00 per thousand

o      STEP 2 - Multiply rate times the tax base (taxable value) to obtain
       the tax levy.
       Example: $85,825,932

o      STEP 3 - Multiply the levy by .95 in order to compensate for
       noncollection of some taxes. The result is the amount of property
       revenue which can be budgeted for the forthcoming fiscal year.
       Example: $81,534,635
```

on property that would normally be taxed. Of critical concern to many taxpayers in Florida is the fact that homeowner-residents are entitled to a homestead exemption of $25,000 dollars for their principal residence. Thus, a home appraised at $105,000 is actually taxed at $80,000. Finally, underassessments have the impact of exempting real value from taxation. After the full value of all property is determined and all exemptions have been subtracted, the remainder is the property tax base for the county. Across the state of Florida, roughly two-thirds of the full valuation of property is *not* part of this tax base due to the three reasons cited above. While the exact percentage varies across states and locales, the magnitude of property values excluded from taxation is commonly very high.

Step Three—Calculations

After exemptions are applied, the taxable value of property has been determined. The sum of the taxable value of all property within its boundaries constitutes the tax base for a local government. Once the tax base is known, the tax rate can be determined (see Exhibit 7-4 for definitions of terms and concepts critical to the rate-setting process).

Calculation of the property tax is a relatively simple matter, but it can be approached in two different ways. The two methods will be demonstrated using the data from Exhibit 7-3.

In the first method, the local government decides how much money it wishes to obtain from the property tax, a figure known as the tax levy. This amount is then divided by the tax base to determine the tax rate. Since the rate is usually expressed in terms of mills (1/1000 of a dollar), the result of dividing the levy by the base is then multiplied by 1000 to express the rate as tax dollars due per $1000 of assessed valuation (see Exhibit 7-5).

The second method of calculating the property tax assumes that local officials first determine the rate which they wish to authorize. The rate is then multiplied by the tax base to determine the levy, which is the amount of property tax revenue the government will have available to spend in the coming fiscal year (see Exhibit 7-6).

In a growing area like the one considered in our example here, the tax base may increase substantially in a single year. In our sample government, the tax base grew from $18,379,211,772 to $21,456,483,992, an increase of over $3 billion, or roughly a 17% gain. **This change is the result of two factors: the increased value of existing property due to reassessment and the worth of new construction.** These components provide an opportunity to increase property tax revenues without changing the tax rate. For instance, since the tax base here has increased about 17%, the government can claim that it has not increased taxes by keeping its tax rate the same as last year, but still collect 17% more in taxes.

94   PRACTICAL GOVERNMENT BUDGETING

Exhibit 7-7   The Revenue Impact of Property Value Changes

The calculations of property value changes and their impact on tax rates and revenues under Florida's TRIM law provide insight into the property tax for managers everywhere. The process is as follows:

o   STEP 1 - Begin with the prior year tax levy, which was the result of the prior year tax rate multiplied by the prior year taxable value.
    Example: $72,256,033

o   STEP 2 - The total change in the tax base (current year taxable value minus prior year taxable value) is reduced by the value of new construction to determine the current year adjusted value (the new value of the prior year tax base after annual reassessment).
    Example: $20,153,255,177

o   STEP 3 - Divide Step 1 total by Step 2 total to give the tax rate which would produce exactly the same tax levy this year as last year on the same property. This rate is called the rollback rate. In this example, the current year rate will be less than the prior year rate of 3.9314 since the existing tax base has increased in value.
    Example: $3.5853 per thousand

o   STEP 4 - The rollback rate of $3.5853 is then multiplied times the value of new construction, and this result is added to the prior year levy to establish the total amount of taxes which may be levied without advertising a tax increase to the citizens. Alternatively, the rollback rate could simply be multiplied by the total current year taxable value. The result is the same.
    Example: $76,927,932

o   NOTE - The tax base for the next fiscal year's revenues is the current year taxable value.

o   NOTE - Determining and correcting for noncollection of taxes at .95% is not included in these calculations of rollback rates and resulting levies. If a local government anticipated a rise in uncollected taxes, it would have to increase its tax rate beyond the rollback rate in order to compensate.

Such action cannot escape notice in Florida due to the state's Truth in Millage (TRIM) law. Under the TRIM law, governments must determine the tax rate which would generate the same total revenues (proceeds) as were levied in the past year on the same property. This is called the rollback rate. Any proposed tax rate higher than the rollback rate requires localities to notify taxpayers that a tax increase is being proposed. The concept is that governments should not be allowed to capture the increase in the value of property without notifying citizens that there is an increase in taxes (see Exhibit 7-7).

New construction is excluded from these calculations because new construction may well require new services from the government. Thus taxing new construction at the rollback rate is considered to be keeping taxes level.

Florida's TRIM law imposes a set of unique notification procedures on its local governments. Moreover, the logic behind it is a bit flawed since increases in assessed value of property are often less than the increases in the cost of providing public services. Still, the TRIM law helps us understand the property tax better and it is quite useful for local officials and managers everywhere to be able to dissect the tax carefully and explain its components. It is important to understand the revenue and expenditure implications of changes in the value of existing property plus the impact of any new additions to the tax base.

Step Four—Collection

Procedures for collecting the property tax vary from place to place, but are often the responsibility of an elected Tax Collector. In our Florida example, the Tax Collector is an elected county official who executes the collection process for all property taxing bodies in the county, which include the county itself, cities, schools, and special districts. Once each government has determined its tax rate, the Collector prepares tax bills for every piece of property in the county. This is done by accumulating the individual goverment tax rates into a total rate and multiplying that times the value of each parcel of property. Since the cities and special districts have various and overlapping boundaries, there are many different taxing areas within a single county. Each is served by a unique combination of local governments, each is identified by its own millage code, and each has its distinct **total** tax rate.

Prompt payment of taxes is stimulated by a system of discounts for early payment and interest penalties for late payment. The ultimate penalty for nonpayment is seizure and sale of property by the Collector, an option which is approached with the utmost caution and elaborate procedures by an elected official. Still, the nature of the property tax makes it one of the easiest to collect for governments. Therefore, governments can usually depend on collecting most of the tax levied. A common practice is to budget collections at 95% of the total levy. This is a state-imposed requirement in Florida, and is likely a safe margin for local governments everywhere unless they serve communities experiencing economic hardships.

Three Perspectives on the Property Tax

Elected officials, taxpaying citizens, and local government agency administrators view the property tax from distinctive points of view. Public managers need to appreciate the differences between their own outlook and those of elected officials and taxpayers. They also need to be able to communicate their agency needs in terms of these other perspectives.

The annual decision on the property tax rate is usually the most significant and visible action taken by elected officials each year. **Two conflicting needs must be reconciled: the projected budgetary expenditures needed to provide services versus the desire to keep the unpopular property tax to a minimum.** In terms of meeting budget needs, the property tax is something of a blessing because it is a major source of income and the amount to be collected can be easily adjusted in the normal workings of the budget process. Few, if any, other revenue sources available to local governments are both open to local rate changes and capable of producing dollars anywhere near those of the property tax. Unless a government is taxing at or near a state-imposed limitation (10 mills in Florida), the legal authority to increase the rate exists in the budget adoption process. Therefore, many local governments do in fact determine budgetary needs, substract all other sources of revenue, and use the property tax to secure the difference. This can be considered "bottom-up" budgeting, since spending needs drive the determination of the tax rate (see Method 1 in Exhibit 7-5).

On the other hand, elected officials must be cognizant of the impact of the tax levy on the tax rate. For many citizens and elected officials themselves it is the bottom line function of government to be frugal and efficient. Holding the line on the tax rate constitutes the most easily available measure of success. If local officials first reach agreement on a tax rate and then approve only those budget

Exhibit 7-8   A Property Tax Bill

A. 1985 TAX NOTICE/RECEIPT   COUNTY REAL ESTATE TAXES

	NOV 4%	DEC 3%	JAN 2%	FEB 1%	MAR
	184.56	189.61	194.56	499.70	504.75

CHECKS PAYABLE

TAX COLLECTOR

EX-TYPE	ESCROW CODE	MILLAGE CODE
		58

B.

ASSESSED VALUES

TAXES LEVIED

COUNTY	108.86
SCHOOL	159.80
LIBRY	13.48
SPEC PUR	31.78
HX 25,000	SFWM	9.63
EE EX	FIRE U	58.56
WD EX	UTD	18.84
NEX 21,942	MST/G	103.80
TOT   46,942

ACCT 999999-9

DOE JOHN J
& PATTY F
1027 N SMITH ST
ANYTOWN FL 32800

C.

D.&H.

E. 22 22 30 4300 02061

F. CROSBY ADD N YOUNG SUB T/66

G. CLK 2 LOT 6

0726/1592
(PLEASE TURN OVER) THIS TAX NOTICE BECOMES A RECEIPT WHEN VALIDATED BY TAX COLLECTOR

PAID   123********7,3*0, 484.56 NOV 2, 85 01

0090012015022050025015021000

A. **Total Tax Due** - (March) Discount given if paid earlier. 4%-November; 3%-December and 1% February.

B. **Millage Code** - See millage chart for corresponding number indicated on tax bill-shows tax rates for your area.

C. **Taxable Value** - Tax rates applied to this value.

D. **MST** - Municipal Service Taxing Unit (Service Charges) example: lights, retention pond, etc.

E. **Taxes Levied** - After applying tax rate to taxable value.

F. **Legal Description.**

G. **After Payment** - Validation area: Receipt number; amount and date paid.

H. **Note:** The Taxes Levied column - If indicated as MST-G: you are being charged for garbage collection.

Exhibit 7-9   Communicating with the Taxpayer

```
                    MILLAGE AND TAXES
                   Average City Homeowner
                    Fiscal Year 1986/87

          Taxable Value of Average Home = $35,000
```

Government	Millage	Taxes Due	% of Total
County	3.911	$136.89	27%
School	7.375	$258.12	50%
Library	1.000	$35.00	7%
Other Special Districts	.515	$18.02	3%
Special Levy	.500	$17.50	3%
City	1.414	$49.49	10%
TOTALS	14.715	$515.02	100%

requests which fit within the revenues generated by that rate, this is called the "top-down" approach (see Method 2 in Exhibit 7-6).

In fact, elected officials typically look at proposed budget expenditures in terms of implications for the tax rate and then consider what different tax rates would permit in terms of spending. Thus **there is usually a back-and-forth analysis which includes both "top-down" and "bottom-up" considerations.** Obviously, upcoming elections, public sentiment about taxes, and the severity of public needs for spending shape the application of elected officials' philosophies and attitudes about the needs of spending versus taxing. Some years the perceived need to limit the tax rate will be the predominant consideration. In other years, the desire to maintain, improve, or expand services will be the highest priority.

For the taxpayer, the property tax is a big confusing bill. Taxpayers rarely know where the money is going or what it pays for (see Exhibit 7-8). When the tax bill is taken apart and related to specific services, the costs may be much smaller and more reasonable. However, a single large bill listing only the names of governmental units and their tax rates is not usually received with pleasure. Since most taxpayers have little knowledge or contact with the local governments which serve them, the receipt of a tax bill may be their major experience with the taxing body. If they do use one or more services, they may well take the position that "Service X" is fine, but everything else should be cut back to keep rates down.

Public managers, therefore, should be acutely aware of the relationship between their agency budget and the property tax. Alternative revenue sources should be identified and developed whenever possible, thus enhancing the chances that their budget requests will be approved. Where reliance on the property tax revenues is necessary, the degree of dependence should be precisely documented, ideally in terms of service units, and translated into the perspectives of elected officials (what do the additional funds we are requesting mean for the tax rate?) and citizens (what do those new funds mean for your property tax bill?). Exhibit 7-9 provides an example, at the municipal level, of this communication process, intended to inform citizens of the small portion of their total tax bill which goes for city services. It can be valuable to carry this presentation the additional steps just suggested. For instance, in the city just described it costs the average city homeowner $26 per year or $.50 per week for municipal police service. When taxes and services are expressed in these terms, taxpayers may gain new insights and adopt new attitudes about the property tax and the services it supports.

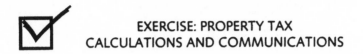

EXERCISE: PROPERTY TAX CALCULATIONS AND COMMUNICATIONS

1. Read the following and respond to the questions:

On July 1, the Property Appraiser certified a tax roll which shows evidence of continued growth and development throughout the county. Current taxable valuation has grown to $15.8 billion. This represents a 23.2% increase over last year's taxable valuation of $12.8 billion. Of this approximate $3 billion increase in taxable valuation, 1.1 billion (37.6%) is attributable to new construction while $1.9 billion (62.4%) of the increase is attributable to reassessments.

The proposed county government budget for upcoming Fiscal Year 1991-1992 anticipates a millage of 4.9611. This represents an increase of .8445 mills (+20.5%) over the FY 1990-1991 rate of 4.1166 mills.

   a. What is the proposed tax levy for Fsical Year 1991-1992?

   b. What is the roll back tax rate for Fiscal Year 1991-1992?

   c. What would the tax levy be if the roll back rate were adopted instead of the proposed tax rate?

   d. What is the exact difference between the revenues the county should budget if it adopts the proposed rate versus the roll back rate?

   e. What difference would the choice between the proposed and the roll back rate make in the tax bill for the owner-occupants of a home assessed at $125,000?

2. Review the data below and perform the requested calculations. Assume that "taxes" consist entirely of property taxes, that the total tax base is $18,750,000,000, that the average home has a taxable value of $130,000, and that 100% of taxes levied are collected.

Fiscal Year 1988-1989
Sources of Revenue
for Program Expenditures

| | PROGRAMS | | |
Revenues	Emergency 911	Highway Maintenance	Recreation & Parks
Taxes	$ 863,285	$ 665,348	$ 1,383,080
Grants	0	$ 2,652,182	$ 290,450
User Charges	0	0	$ 640,100
Revenue Bonds	0	$ 11,026,973	0
TOTAL	$ 863,285	$ 14,344,503	$ 2,313,630

a. What will the average homeowner pay in property taxes to fund FY88-89 services for the three programs listed in the Table?

b. Assume that the City Council has "suggested" that the Recreation and Parks Department fund 50% of its budget (exclusive of grants) from user charges. Using the data in the table and assuming that 87,500 user charge fees will be collected **regardless** of the amount of the user fee, answer the following questions:

   - How much will the tax rate be reduced?
   - How much will the average homeowner save on the property tax bill?
   - What will be the increase in the average user charge?

c. If the Emergency-911 Program adds an Assistant Program Director at a **total** annual cost of $54,500, how much will this impact the tax rate? How much will the average homeowner's tax bill increase?

100

Chapter 8

THE CAPITAL BUDGET PROCESS _____

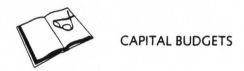

CAPITAL BUDGETS

HOW THIS CHAPTER WILL BE USEFUL

In previous chapters, we discussed how an agency would develop its budget to include expenditures for capital outlay as well as personal services and operating expenses. These smaller capital expenditures, such as rolling stock, office furniture, and equipment, generally are part of the agency's operating budget. This chapter will discuss larger local government capital expenditures such as land acquisition or construction of public buildings that are normally included in a **capital budget**.

The capital budget is the first and current year of a local government's Five-year **Capital Improvement Program (CIP)**, which details the government entity's long-range capital improvement needs. In order to understand a local government's capital budget, one should be familiar with the terms and concepts in Exhibit 8-1.

After becoming aware of the time-consuming and tedious process that is associated with developing an operating budget, you might ask yourself: Why have **another** budget process specifically for major capital improvement projects? The intention is that these very expensive, long-term commitments be given very special attention.

Therefore, governments commonly establish a uniform and organized five year **Capital Improvement Program (CIP)** to outline the public facilities, infrastructure, and land purchases that the jurisdiction intends to implement during a multi-year period, given the estimated funds available for financing these projects. The CIP is generally revised on an annual basis and the **first year** included in the current plan is a mirror image of that fiscal year's **Capital Budget**. This systematic review of proposed projects affords the jurisdiction the opportunity to tie all these major, costly

Exhibit 8-1   Capital Budget Terms and Concepts

Capital Budget: The capital budget may be a separate document or included as a separate capital improvement section along with the annual operating budget. It is composed of the local government's capital improvements which are major, nonrecurring expenditures, or any significant expenditures for physical facilities.

Capital Improvement: Capital improvements are any major, nonrecurring expenditures for physical facilities of a government that result in the acquisition of an addition to the fixed assets. This includes items such as land acquisition, construction/renovation of buildings or other structures, or other improvements that could include the construction of roads, a water and sewer system, or a ball field. Capital improvements normally have a useful life of 5 years or more. The dollar limitation on classifying a project as a "capital improvement" varies in each jurisdiction. However, projects of $25,000 or more are often considered to be "capital improvements."

Capital Improvement Program (CIP): The CIP is the long-range schedule of capital improvement projects with their estimated costs, normally for a 5 year period. This includes a 4 year period beyond the capital improvement budget for the current fiscal year.

---

projects together with respect to scheduling/timing, location, and financing. This review should result in the logical development, construction, and funding of projects.

A significant element of planning the multi-year CIP and the fiscal year's Capital Budget is the financial analysis aimed at minimizing the impact of the projects on the local tax rate, while maximizing the "power" of dollars available for the projects. The capital budget process, therefore, is not only a management tool for guiding the expenditure of public resources over an extended period of time, but also represents a commitment by the local government to provide its community with the desired, and required, level of service.

OBJECTIVES

Upon completing this chapter, the reader should be able to perform the following tasks:

1. Describe the importance of preparing a separate capital budget.

2. Define capital budget, capital improvement, and capital improvement program (CIP) and discuss how they interrelate.

3. Discuss the steps involved in the capital budget process.

4. Describe the major funding mechanisms utilized by local governments to finance their capital improvement projects.

 PREPARING CAPITAL BUDGETS

The **Techniques** section of this chapter will discuss four separate areas of the capital budget process. They are as follows:

- Components of the Capital Budget
- Pros and Cons of Capital Budgeting
- Developing a Capital Budget
- Financing Capital Improvements

Components of the Capital Budget

In Chapter 4, we discussed how to prepare an agency's operating and capital outlay requests. The term "capital outlay" utilized in Chapter 4 refers to capital expenditures for items such as vehicles, office furniture, or equipment. Chapter 8 also refers to "capital outlay" items but holds a different connotation since it is associated with a capital **not operating** budget. A. John Vogt, describes capital outlay in the following manner:

> Capital outlays are durable—that is, they yield benefits for many years, or they result in the acquisition of property that has a long life. Capital outlays do not usually recur each year, . . . and are also typically expensive, requiring large expenditures.[1]

Exhibit 8-2   Careful CIP Planning for all Future Contingencies

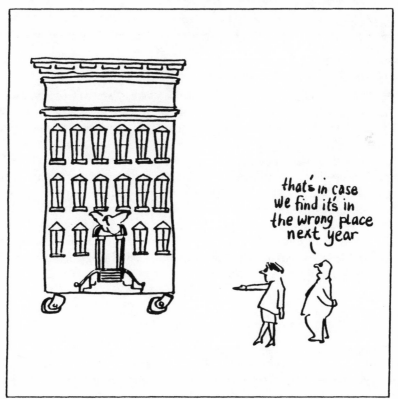

Exhibit 8-3   What Is Included in the Capital Budget?

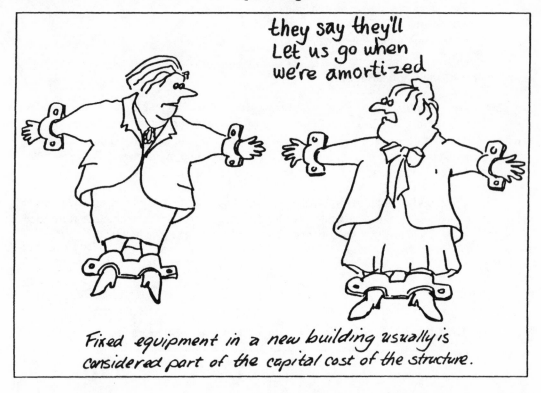

Fixed equipment in a new building usually is considered part of the capital cost of the structure.

Therefore, when referring to capital outlay in this chapter, we will be discussing durable, nonrecurring, typically expensive acquisitions. This would include items such as land purchases, building construction/renovation, or other improvements such as water and sewer systems, road construction, or ball fields.

Each governmental jurisdiction has a dollar limit that separates capital outlay items that it considers as part of the operating budget from those placed in the capital budget. This amount would vary depending upon the local government and its interpretation of the definition of a capital budget and capital improvement project. In any case, however, a capital budget **should not** include any capital outlay that may meet the dollar limit of a capital budget item but **recurs** on an annual basis. Such an example would be the routine, annual replacement of the Fire Department's fire apparatus. These items are considered to be part of the normal operating costs of the Department and, therefore, should be included in the annual operating budget.

Advantages and Disadvantages

As stated earlier, a Capital Improvement Program represents the budget year's improvements and an orderly schedule for improvements four years or so into the future. Some important advantages that a capital budget may provide a local government are:[2]

- Prevents duplication of projects and equipment
- Provides a vehicle for coordinating projects
- Establishes project priorities
- Helps provide for an equitable distribution of public improvements throughout the community
- Allows maximum benefits from available public funds
- Coordinates the physical and the financial planning of projects
- Provides citizens and management with information on short- and long-range projects and their potential costs

It should be emphasized that probably the most important aspect of capital improvement budgets is that they give the local government a mechanism for long-range physical and fiscal planning. It is very easy for local governments to sit down and develop a "wish list" of projects they'd like to complete. However, in reality, if monies are not available to fund the projects, then the list is of no value.

Capital improvement budgeting is definitely an effective management tool to be utilized by local governments in making budget decisions. However, there are some problems associated with capital budgeting. The first problem encountered is that the capital budgeting process **assumes** that

Exhibit 8-4   CIP Programming Calendar

January 1-31	Coordinating unit prepares inventory of current facilities
February 1-28	All appropriate persons identify possible projects
March 1-31	Planning body comments on all projects
April 1-30	Coordinating unit prepares six-year schedule of projects and makes decisions on methods of financing based on financial analysis
April 15-May 15	Public Hearings held
May 1-June 15	Draft CIP finalized and projects scheduled for upcoming year are incorporated into annual budget
June 1-June 15	Legislative body consideration and review of six-year schedule and one-year capital budget
June 15	CIP and first year budget is adopted, followed by preparation, review, and establishment of acquisition and development plans
July 1	Beginning of fiscal year

there will be a continuous cycle of reappraisal and reevaluation of project proposals. This seems like an obvious part of the process since community needs change from year to year. These changes may be based on an area's growth or even shifts in the political climate of the community. Often times, however, CIP's are developed, printed, and distributed and never reviewed after that. The CIP may be followed blindly or, in the opposite case, may be modified without the kind of full review that led to the initial development of the CIP. To avoid these problems, a continuous review of the CIP is important in insuring that the community's needs are, and will be, met.

Second, there is the universal problem determining which projects are **truly** capital improvements program material. For example, an item to be purchased may meet capital budget project dollar limits. However, due to the need for recurring purchases of this particular very expensive item, it could also be considered as an operating budget item. The interpretation of "capital outlay" for the CIP often varies from jurisdiction to jurisdiction.

Third, the availability of funds often distorts the ranking of projects. Some projects have their own funding source which makes them seem more "attractive" or feasible. Monies may be earmarked for specific projects, such as gas tax dollars for use only on road projects, or a project may be "revenue producing," such as a water and sewer system. This often enables these projects to forgo the "possible funding source" problem faced by the other projects. This factor should not exempt such projects from receiving the same review and analysis as other projects when determining their feasibility and appropriateness.

Finally, there is the pressing problem in deciding which projects are the **most** important. In making these decisions, one should objectively consider those projects that benefit the community the most. However, here too the proverbial problems of funding availability and political climate come into consideration.

Developing a Capital Budget

The process involved in actually developing a capital budget entails the cooperation and input of many "players" in the local government. However, there is normally one agency responsible for coordinating the process. This could be a Planning Department, Budget Office, Development Coordination Bureau, or even a formalized Capital Facilities/Improvements Agency.

Exhibit 8-5   Capital Facilities Inventory

Facility	Replace Cost	Built or Acquired	Condition	Use
Municipal Complex	$7200000	1982	Good	Heavy
Pub Safety Bldg	4500000	1983	Fair	Heavy
Fire Station #1	860000	1976	Fair	Mod
Fire Station #2	630000	1979	Good	Mod
Swimming Pool	440000	1984	Poor	Seasonal
Recreation Center	975000	1981	Exc	Light
Alford Park	2500000	1971	Good	Mod
Ashe Park	1100000	1978	Good	Mod

PRACTICAL GOVERNMENT BUDGETING

Exhibit 8-6   Considering Future Capital Needs

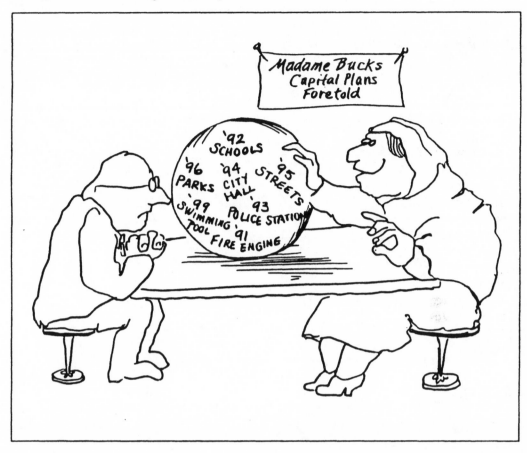

The actual capital budget process varies with each local jurisdiction. However, there are three distinct stages that all processes adhere to: planning, budget, and implementation.

In the **planning** stage, the local government must first develop a CIP programming calendar which highlights critical dates in the CIP process (Exhibit 8-4).[3] The calendar is useful in coordinating the work of all the "players" and identifies "who does what, and when?" during the process. It also ensures that each step is accomplished so that the process may continue in a timely and efficient manner.

The next crucial step in the planning stage is to develop an inventory of existing facilities. This will facilitate in determining the need for the renewal, replacement, expansion, or even retirement of current inventory. Exhibit 8-5,[4] Capital Facilities Inventory, provides a sample format that could be utilized to assess a jurisdiction's existing facilities. This information can be obtained from a current fixed asset inventory list or building records for insurance tcoverage. Once a list has been compiled, all agency heads should review it to ensure that all existing public facilities and improvements are included and accurately described.

The next step in the planning stage is to determine the status of previously approved CIP projects. Compilation of this information is important in that it identifies which projects are being

Exhibit 8-7 Capital Project Request Form

This form must be completed for each Capital Project to include construction, repair, or modifications.

(1) Title of Project: Renovation to Heather Brook Fire Station

(2) Location: Heather Brook, Ocean County

Description and Justification: Specify details concerning the nature of the project and reasons it is required.

Improvements to this Fire Station are needed due to the increased activity in this quadrant. The opening of the Heather Brook subdivision makes it mandatory that the County be able to respond to calls in this area in an efficient and effective manner. Renovations to this station will include expanding (1) the existing bay area capability from 2 to 3 fire apparatus vehicles; (2) the sleeping quarters to accomodate an additional 10 fire personnel; and (3) the kitchen area.

ESTIMATED COST OF PROJECT

PROJECT COST COMPONENTS:		PROJECT ANNUAL COSTS:	
Land,ROW	$ 0	1st Year	$ 60,000
Design	$ 60,000	2nd Year	$ 350,000
Construction	$ 250,000	3rd Year	$
Repair/Mod.	$	4th Year	$
Equipment	$ 100,000	5th Year	$
Other Costs	$	TOTAL	$ 410,000

CURRENT STATUS OF PROJECT: Project has not been implemented to date.

Estimated Project Life: 15 years

Project Source of Funding: GO Bonds

continued, how much money has been expended to date on the project, and what additional funds, if any, are required to complete the project. This report also provides the staff and legislature with information on projects approved in prior years.

Once the organization has identified the status of its previously approved projects, it must determine the future needs of the community. In order to accomplish this task, the CIP coordinating agency provides all agencies with a Capital Project Request Form (Exhibit 8-7) and accompanying instructions on how to complete the form (Exhibit 8-8). The purpose of this form is to obtain input from all governmental agencies in order to assess their long-range capital improvement requirements.

Upon receiving all the requests, a CIP review committee screens and evaluates these requests. Criteria normally used in evaluating the "importance" of a project include the following:

- Degree of urgency of the project
- Benefits derived from the project
- Cost and tax rate impact
- Acceptability to voters

Exhibit 8-8   Instructions for Completing Capital Project Form

```
Detailed instructions for completing this form are as follows:

(1) Title of Project - specify the name of the proposed project.

(2) Location - identify the location of the project, i.e., street address
or other location of the project.

(3) Description and Justification - provide complete description of the
proposed project and specify why the project is needed. Include any results
from project analysis already performed related to the project. Also
indicate the short- and long-range effects on the operating budget.

(4) Estimated Cost of Project - itemize all anticipated expenditures of the
project including land, right-of-way (ROW) fees, construction costs, repair
or modification costs, as well as equipment costs. Also indicate if funds
will be required beyond the first year of the project.

(5) Other Supporting Information - indicate (a) the current status of the
project, i.e., project not yet begun, design completed, land or ROW
purchased,etc; (b) estimated useful life of the project; and (c) the
proposed source of funding for the project such as GO bonds, available cash,
short-term financing.
```

After its review of the project requests, the committee prepares a list of proposed recommended CIP projects and ranks them according to importance and urgency.

In the **budget** stage, the committee must investigate the financing options and the fiscal feasibility of funding the various project requests. The development of the desired capital improvement projects is relatively easy when compared with the task of "finding the money" to finance the projects. There are several options available to local governments as they attempt to accomplish this painful task. Evaluation may be performed by the in-house staff or by a professional engineer or consulting firm.

The number of public improvements that a local government can finance generally depends on: (1) the level of recurring future operating expenditures; (2) the current level of debt (bonded indebtedness); (3) the legal limit of debt it may incur (bonded capacity); and (4) any potential sources of additional revenue available for capital improvement financing.[5] Upon taking these items into consideration, the committee must then select the most appropriate financing mechanism available for each project.

One excellent method is that of **pay-as-you-go** which means financing capital with current revenues. In other words, pay in cash. This is an option that we as individuals would like to have but can rarely afford when making major purchases such as buying an automobile, putting in a swimming pool, or adding another room to our home. This method can work well for governmental jurisdictions when the capital needs are small and surplus revenues are available. The major advantage to utilizing this funding alternative is that it saves on costs (interest rates, repayment schedules, closing fees, and bond issuance expenses) that are associated with borrowing money to finance the project.

Despite its desirable qualities, the pay-as-you-go method is by no means infallible. One of the criticisms of this method is that the existing population is paying for projects that future generations will enjoy and benefit from. The local government is also depleting its available cash reserves on projects that could easily be financed, thereby spreading payments over many years.

A second, and very popular, financing alternative is that of **issuing bonds** for the construction of capital improvement projects. This method is particularly feasible when the project has a long, useful life, such as a building, water and sewer plant, or roads, or can be financed by service charges to pay off revenue bonds. The process of securing and issuing bonds, however, can be very costly and time-consuming. It also involves working with bond counsel in order to obtain their expert advice on issuing bonds.

In dealing with bond issuance, there are normally two kinds of bonds which local governments seek: General Obligation (GO) Bonds and revenue bonds. GO bonds are usually limited by state law as to the amount, as well as the length, of indebtedness that a government can have. These "full faith and credit" bonds are secured by all of the financial assets of the local government, including property taxes. Demographic and economic information, as well as a local government's fiscal condition, are all considered in determining the "risk" involved in providing GO bonds for projects. The second type of bond normally issued is called revenue bonds. These bonds are used for the purchase or construction of public facilities that produce revenue such as toll roads. The local government must repay the debt from revenue produced by the facility over a specified number of years.

A third method of financing capital improvements is that of **securing short-term notes or using a line of credit (LOC).** In this method a substantial amount of money is made available for the local government to utilize on an "as needed" basis. The money, when used, is then repaid in installments over the next few years at a predetermined, normally desirable, interest rate. This funding alternative is helpful for both the local government and the lending institution. The local government has access to the money as it is needed, while the lending institution has a "trustworthy and reliable" customer.

A final funding mechanism that is utilized by local governments is **joint financing**. This situation occurs when cities and counties jointly finance a project, such as an administration office building or recreational complex. The exact funding alternative used is normally determined by agreement of the different jurisdictions involved in the process. This is a desirable method in that it shifts the financial burden and obligation to more than one local government.

A summary of selected projects and their funding sources such as Exhibit 8-9[6] is then developed and submitted to the Chief Executive and/or the Legislature for their review. In addition, forms such as shown in Exhibit 8-10 are prepared to detail each project as submitted to the legislative body as part of a CIP document. Note that this information includes the project description, history, future years' estimated costs, and also the dollars spent on the project in prior years.

In the final **implementation** stage, formal adoption of the capital budget occurs. A copy of the proposed five year CIP including the proposed capital budget for the next fiscal year should be provided to the legislative body prior to any formal discussions/workshops. This allows time for each legislator to examine each of the proposed projects being recommended and formulate any questions they might have regarding the project proposals. For the legislative body, the CIP is an important management tool in that it:

- Allows them to be better informed on the need for large capital expenditures on a short- and long-term basis
- Forces them to consider, and make recommendations on, the future capital improvements for the community
- Helps inform the citizenry of the jurisdiction's intent, for the next five years, to acquire and/or develop capital facilities in the community.

Exhibit 8-9   Summary of Selected CIP Projects

Project	Cost	1984	1985	1986	1987	1988	FS	Pay Sch
Pub Wks Equip	60000	4400	4400	4400	4400	4400	GO	15 yrs
Remodel Fire St	700000	51000	51000	51000	51000	51000	GO	15 yrs
Water Well #6	200000				14000	14000	RB	15 yrs
Water Well #7	200000					14000	RB	15 yrs
Storm Sewer #53	120000	8000	8000	8000	8000	8000	SAB	15 yrs
Swim Pool	55000	55000					GF	1 yr
Lee Avenue Widen	476000	238000	238000				SHA	2 yrs
Campbell Rd Ext	750000			250000	250000	250000	SHA	3 yrs
Park Land Acq	950000	190000	190000	190000	190000	190000	LCF	5 yrs
Totals	2761000	546400	491400	503400	517400	531400		

```
GO  - General Obligation Bond
RB  - Revenue Bond
SAB - Special Assessment Bond
GF  - General Fund
SHA - State Highway Aid
LCF - Land Conservation Fund
```

To approve the CIP, the normal procedure is to adopt the first year of the proposed CIP, the capital budget, and incorporate this as a separate portion of the annual operating budget. The remaining four years of the program is usually accepted by resolution, subject to annual revision and authorization. The acceptance of the five year plan is not binding since it is subject to future legislative body scrutiny.

Exhibit 8-10   Agency CIP Summary

Division:	County Administration
Project:	Oak Street Building Renovation
Description:	In FY 1985-86, the County acquired this 87,000 square foot building to relieve overcrowding in existing facilities. After renovation, all Tax, Records, and Data Services will be relocated to this facility.
Funding:	Proceeds from 1986 Sales Tax Revenue Bonds.

Funding by Fiscal Year

Total Cost	FY87-88	FY88-89	FY89-90	FY90-91	FY91-92
$3684000	$420000	$1966000	$1298000	0	0

Upon approval, the proper steps are taken to actually acquire and expend the funds to implement the approved capital projects. This is the point where bonds are issued or other financing secured. Once the fiscal arrangements have been properly addressed, then the local government may proceed in actually acquiring land for the new library facility or hiring a firm to design the new water and sewer plant or otherwise begin whatever projects have been accepted. The three stages identified above constitute a full and complete capital budget process.

Conclusion

As described in this chapter, the preparation of a capital budget involves an intricate process. However, it does focus special attention on major expenditures. The end result proves to be not only a management tool for guiding the expenditure of public resources over a period of time, but also represents a commitment by the local government to acquire, construct, and maintain adequate physical facilities to provide the desired, and required, level of service to its community.

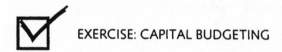 EXERCISE: CAPITAL BUDGETING

1. The city of Oceanside is situated on the east coast and currently has a population of 30,000. In the Fall of 1992, the Merrimac Defense Plan will open for full operation. The plan currently has a work force of 200 but this number will soon grow to 1000 employees. The availability of jobs at the plant has resulted in tremendous growth in population north of the city limits where the plant is located. Many people are moving to the Heather Brook subdivision which is approximately 5 miles from the plant. The subdivision, located on US15, is 55% developed now.

There are currently two capital improvement problems that Oceanside must address. First, US15, north of the city, needs to be widened to four lanes. This improvement is needed in order to handle the increased traffic related to the opening of the Merrimac Defense Plan, as well as the expansion of the Heather Brook subdivision. The road-widening project will take at least three years to complete. The Federal Transportation Department will finance 80% of the costs to widen the road. Second, the city must replace the aging main station of its water and sewer system.

The fiscal state of the city is such that it will be able to appropriate only $1,000,000 per year for capital improvements. Therefore, projects must be prioritized and consideration given to those items that could be classified as part of the operating budget. **The data presented here, along with departmental project proposals detailed below, is to be used to prepare a capital improvement program for the years 1990 to 1994 and a capital budget for 1990.**

The following projects have been proposed by the city of Oceanside department heads:

Water and Sewer Department

- Lift Station, Heather Brook—1992, $725,000.
- Storm Sewer Installation, Heather Brook—1993, $850,000.
- Water and Sewer System Replacement, Main Station—1990, $1,500,000.

Transportation/Traffic Engineering Department

- US15 Road Widening—1990, $750,000; 1991, $550,000 (costs are project totals by year).

112

- Curbing/Sidewalks, Heather Brook—1900, $500,000; 1991, $50,000; 1992, $200,000.
- Traffic Signal Repair—1990 to 1998, $35,000 each year.

Fire Services Department

- New Fire Station—1993, $450,000; 1994, $65,000.
- Fire Apparatus:
    - (a) Pumper (main station)—1990, $130,000.
    - (b) Tanker (substation)—1992, $135,000.

Leisure Services Department

- New Library—1991, $2,500,000 (costs for construction, furniture, fixtures, books, parking lot).
- Sweetwater Park Recreation Complex—1991, $35,000; 1992, $125,000; 1993, $225,000; 1994, $95,000.

Your task for this exercise is to prepare a 5 Year Capital Improvement Program (CIP) and a capital budget for the year 1990, as described in paragraph 3 **(in bold type).** All necessary information to accomplish this task is provided above.

NOTES

1. A. John Vogt, "Budgeting Capital Outlays and Improvements," in Jack Rabin *et al.*, editors, *Budget Management* (Athens, Georgia: Carl Vinson Institute of Government, 1983), p. 128.

2. Jack Rabin *et al.*, *Public Budgeting Laboratory Notebook* (Athens, Georgia: Carl Vinson Institute of Government, 1983), p. 45.

3. *A Capital Improvement Programming Handbook* (Chicago, Illinois: Municipal Finance Officers Association, 1978), p. 11.

4. *Capital Budgeting: Blueprints for Change* (Chicago, Illinois: Government Finance Officers Association, 1985), p. 105.

5. *A Capital Improvement Programming Handbook, op. cit.*, p. 18.

6. *Capital Budgeting: Blueprints for Change, op. cit.*, p. 159.

Chapter 9

HOW TO SPEND YOUR BUDGET WISELY _____

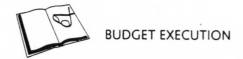 BUDGET EXECUTION

HOW THIS CHAPTER WILL BE USEFUL

The lengthy and complex efforts to develop a local government budget are wasted unless the government uses the approved budget to guide its spending over the course of the fiscal year.

The budget, as approved by the legislative body, is a legally binding document setting limits on how much can be spent by whom and for what purposes during a specific period of time. The budget is also the source for agency authority to incur obligations and make payments for personnel, materials, supplies, contractual services, and equipment. Thus, the budget document is both an instrument of negative control over what agencies can spend as well as a positive source of funds available to public managers to conduct programs and activities.

However, it would be a serious mistake to overlook the fact that a budget is a plan based on estimates of future revenues and expenditures. As estimates prove to be inaccurate, or unforeseen events affect revenue collection or agency spending, adjustments must be made in the budget plan. No budget is ever executed exactly as planned and adopted.

Therefore, in this chapter we will return to the three major budget goals of control, management, and planning and note how each may be pursued during the budget execution process. In conclusion, we will touch on the topics of accounting and auditing and note how the types and procedures of auditing help us evaluate and improve our pursuit of these three goals.

In this chapter, you should acquire skills and knowledge to enable you to function effectively in the budget execution process. In particular, you should be able to:

1. Describe the basic elements in the budget execution process.

2. Work with allotments and expenditure controls.

3. Point out the implications of spending procedures, purchasing, and cash management for the daily work of an agency and for the local government as a whole.

4. Explain the fundamentals of governmental accounting and auditing.

PLANS, MANAGEMENT, AND CONTROL IN BUDGET EXECUTION

The Stages of Budget Execution

Some budget execution systems are so primitive and elementary that they are barely sufficient to appease an annual review by an outside auditor. Other local governments boast elaborate computer-based systems utilizing financial, managerial, and cost accounting techniques. These systems allow officials to monitor, adjust, and control spending; maximize effectiveness and efficiency; and develop long-term revenue and expenditure strategies.

Unfortunately, despite the existence of Generally Accepted Accounting Principles (GAAP) for governments and the presence of a strong professional organization, the Government Finance Officers Association (GFOA), budget execution practices and terminology vary somewhat among the federal, state, and local governments. The basics, however, almost always include five stages:

- **Authorization** is the law or statute which permits spending for a specified purpose. Governments can only spend money for activities they are legally permitted to carry out.

- **Appropriation** is the legal authority to expend up to a certain amount of funds during the budget period. For most local governments, the annual budget document is the source for all or most appropriations.

- **Allocations** maybe used by the chief executive, central budget office, and even large agencies to provide further detail to the appropriations approved by the city council, county commission, or other local legislative body. For example, lump-sum appropriations to an agency may need to be further divided into allocations for specific programs the agency operates, split among offices within the agency which administer portions of the budget, or even specified as particular allowable objects of expenditure (line items). The basis for such allocations is the initial agency budget requests, adjusted as necessary for the changes in funding levels and input on preferred programs and activities which occurred in the budget review and approval process. (Note that the terms *allocations*, *apportionments*, and even *allotments* may be used for the same procedures by different jurisdictions.)

Exhibit 9-1   A Basic Budget Allotment Procedure

Like most budgeting techniques, an allotment system is a combination of mathematics and professional judgement. It includes four parts: a plan based on budgetary estimates, monitoring actual expenditures, reporting real expenditures compared to the estimates, and making adjustments if necessary. A basic quarterly allotment plan could be developed as follows:

o   **Develop estimates** by gathering data on spending for each quarter in recent years and adjust as necessary. For instance:

 o   Gather spending-by-quarter data for past five years.
 o   Compute the percent of annual spending for each quarter of each year.
 o   Compute average percent spent in each quarter by dividing the total spent in each quarter over the past five years by the grand total spent for five years.
 o   Adjust average percents for clear trends in most recent years.
 o   Apply adjusted quarterly average to current year budget to set allotments by quarter.
 o   Remove dollars associated with any large, planned, unusual spending patterns anticipated in the coming fiscal year from the allotments and then reinsert them as appropriate.

o   **Monitor spending versus estimates** to determine if pattern of spending is consistent with the allotment plan.

o   **Reporting** should be at least quarterly and should show budgeted amounts, expenditures, and encumbrances for the quarter and the year to date, the percent of the budget expended and encumbered to date, and the amount of the budget still available for spending. Reports should compare all of this current year data to the allotment plan.

o   **Adjustments** should be made where necessary depending upon the identification of deviations from the plan and the analysis of the reasons for these deviations. Adjustments may range from clamping down on careless spending to accelerating or even transferring additional funding for necessary spending at a pace or amount not anticipated.

• **Allotments** divide appropriations or allocations, if any, into time periods such as quarters or months of the fiscal year covered by the approved budget. While some agencies may spend money evenly throughout the year, there is a seasonal pattern to many activities. Thus, allotment plans require historical investigation and close consultation on future intentions to determine whether an even or particular type of uneven allotment would be most appropriate for the particular agency (see Exhibits 9-1 and 9-2).[1]

The allotment device is critical to ensuring that spending is carried out according to the budget insofar as is possible. Allotments also help assure that monies are available to fund operations throughout the fiscal year. Finally, the use of allotments provides an "early warning" system when spending does deviate from the plans approved at the beginning of the fiscal year.

Allotments are used in the construction of cash management plans. If a local government can predict its revenue collections and expenditure patterns with some degree of reliability, it can better formulate plans to invest its cash resources from revenues until such time as they are needed to meet expenditure commitments. Cash management is discussed later in this chapter.

Exhibit 9-2   Development and Use of a Sample Allotment Plan

```
                      Quarterly Expenditure Planning

Police Patrol   1st Quarter  2nd Quarter  3rd Quarter  4th Quarter  Total
                 $     %       $     %       $     %       $     %

Historical:

  FY 1983       100   22.0    125   28.0    125   28.0    100   22.0    450
  FY 1984       110   23.0    130   28.0    125   27.0    105   22.0    470
  FY 1985       110   23.5    125   26.0    130   27.0    110   23.5    475
  FY 1986       120   24.0    130   26.0    135   27.0    115   23.0    500
  FY 1987       125   24.0    140   26.0    145   27.0    120   23.0    530

Computed
Average:              23.3          26.8          27.0          22.7

Adjusted
Average:              24.0          26.0          27.0          23.0

FY 1988
Spending
Projection:    144   24.0    156   26.0    162   27.0    138   23.0    600

Adjusted
Base Budget:   132   24.0    143   26.0    149   27.0    126   23.0    550

Est Deviation:   5            12            16            17             50

Final Planned
Expenditures:  137          155           165           143            600
```

```
                     First Quarter Expenditure Report


Police Patrol  Annual Budget  1st Qtr Budget  1st Qtr Actual  Balance
                                $       %        $       %

                  $600        $137   22.8%     $124   20.6%     $476
```

* All numbers represent 000/s of dollars.

• **Adjustments** may be necessary as revenues and/or spending vary from the projections contained in the annual budget document. Procedures for making adjustments vary from government to government, but usually are multi-level. Agencies are allowed freedom to move "their" appropriated funds (up to a certain amount) across some budget categories. The central budget office is permitted to approve some agency requests for changes in excess of the allowed amounts or beyond the permitted categories. Finally, some adjustments in the budget are considered sufficiently major that the legislature itself must act. This may occur on an ad hoc basis or as part of a comprehensive supplemental budget approval process, which usually happens sometime near the final quarter of the fiscal year.

Spending Money

Once an agency has a budget which it can expend, it begins to make decisions to incur obligations. The agency itself does not directly handle cash, write checks, or use credit cards except for minor, petty-cash-type transactions. Instead, spending money typically involves preparation of a voucher of some sort identifying the authority to spend, the agency and individual issuing the voucher, the account from which funds should be drawn, the items to be purchased, and the name and address of the vendor who should receive payment.

All of this information will be checked and certified by the Treasurer or other designated officials before actual payment is made by the Treasurer's office. Finally, the transaction must be recorded properly according to the local government's accounting system. This provides an "audit trail" so that local government financial affairs can be reviewed and approved by external auditors at the end of the fiscal year.

Every local jurisdiction has its own practices within the bounds of state requirements for spending, but the issues are about the same everywhere. Agencies view budgets as a positive resource to be used to accomplish their mission, goals, and objectives. They favor maximum discretion to use dollars as they best see fit, and tend to view both limitations and reporting requirements as wasteful obstacles to getting the job done. Central budget officials see the budget as a series of procedural rules and substantial limits designed to curb the possibilities for waste, fraud, and abuse, and to protect the fiscal health of the local government. Both perspectives have validity, and the balance between them is probably best struck when each side pursues its claims with vigor. Regardless of the balance which emerges in any particular locality, numerous procedural and substantive controls on spending are likely to exist.

Expenditure Controls

Spending money is subject to a great many limitations, constraints, and controls beyond the allocation and allotment procedures just described. In fact, the most fundamental purposes of the budget and government accounting practices which direct the expenditure process are to control spending within proper bounds and to generate a record that public funds have been spent as directed by elected officials acting on behalf of the people. Closely related to this purpose is the need to be sure that expenditures meet the "Caesar's wife" test: they must not only be proper, they must appear proper to voters and taxpayers. Beyond this emphasis on legality and control, the next priority is to maximize the efficiency with which the citizens' money is translated into public services.

Some of the most common and widely practiced techniques utilized to control expenditures are:

- **Line-Item Appropriations** are a basic control device which confines discretion over spending within very narrow and specific bounds. Agencies may only spend for those "objects of expenditure" approved in the budget process. Further, "pre-audits" may be required before funds may be expended for particular purposes or in excess of set amounts. Essentially a pre-audit is a review of an expenditure decision prior to its actual implementation. For instance, actual expenditures for sensitive items such as travel or equipment may require elaborate advance approval procedures even though funds exist in line items for these purposes. This is a costly and time-consuming approach, best restricted to situations in which waste, fraud, or abuse are either genuine or political areas of concern.

- **Unallocated Reserves** are a common technique used by executives acting through the central budget office to be sure that adequate money is available to meet expenditure demands throughout the budget year. For example, the budget office may withhold 5% of an agency's appropriation from its allotment plan as a kind of emergency reserve should there be a revenue shortfall or unanticipated and unavoidable overspending. Control over such contingency or reserved dollars may be a great source of power in a local government.

- **Encumbrances** are funds designated out of appropriations to be spent only for specific purchases. Money may be encumbered for planned purchases at the very beginning of the fiscal year, or as purchase orders are issued or contracts let. The function of encumbering money is simply to guarantee that appropriated dollars will be available to pay bills when due. Monthly or quarterly statements to agencies should show encumbered as well as expended funds so that managers will know how much spending authority remains for the current year. Once money is actually spent, the encumbrance is liquidated.

  A particular problem is the tendency of agencies to attempt to encumber any unspent dollars as the end of the fiscal year approaches. This often occurs because agency authority to spend unencumbered dollars usually lapses when the fiscal year ends and funds revert to the government's general cash reserve accounts. Like all other spending, the year-end rush can include only items included in the agency's budget. Still, these year-end expenditures are viewed with disfavor by the budget office which emphasizes spending only what is absolutely necessary. In any case, the funding for these items is generally reported as "reservations of fund balance" since the actual expenditures occur in the next fiscal year based on spending authority from the previous fiscal year.

- **Position Control** is an important element of budget control intended to make certain that all new personnel are hired only for positions which have been authorized and included in the annual budget. The steps involve compiling a complete list of approved jobs, establishing a pay plan covering all positions, budgeting adequate funds for all approved positions, and hiring only for approved positions. In any local government of reasonable size, some positions may need to be abolished, created, or reclassified during the budget year. Such actions will need to be approved by the central budget office, and perhaps even the legislature, to be sure that the full and long-range fiscal impacts are considered.

- **Ceilings and freezes** constitute a final and most drastic example of controls imposed on the budget execution process. Ceilings impose an arbitrary limit on expenditures for some or all purposes, while freezes represent a prohibition on further spending for some or all purposes. Usually, such measures are utilized only in times of fiscal or political crisis. For instance, a major revenue shortfall might require an across-the-board ceiling on all controllable expenditures at, say, 80% of the original budgeted amount. Another example might be a political scandal involving contracts with outside consultants which leads to a freeze on the further use of outside experts.

Purchasing

In order to acquire the resources necessary to operate government programs, many budget dollars are expended on the purchase of goods and services from the private sector. In fact in 1987, state and local governments spent about $220 billion to acquire commodities and contractual services from private businesses. With so much money at stake, more local governments are moving to a more centralized and professional approach to purchasing. The intentions are not only to avoid corruption and political influence, but also to achieve maximum efficiencies through volume buying and more expert "shopping" skills.

To operating agencies, the growing power of purchasing officials can seem like another source of red tape and delay but there are a number of sound reasons to use such a system. The Model Procurement Code developed by the American Bar Association and the National Association of State Purchasing Officials sets forth the basics of a good system:[2]

- **Centralization** is required to ensure integrity, effectiveness, and efficiency through a standardized process.

- **Competitive bids and/or negotiations** are the preferred process for most situations to guarantee integrity, maintain public and vendor confidence in the purchasing process, and attract the most potential suppliers and the best terms.

- **A Code of Ethics** should be adopted to strictly forbid purchasing officials from accepting anything of value from a potential vendor or from awarding a contract to any firm with which the official has an affiliation.

- **Standard procedures and open records** require careful and accessible documentation of all purchasing decisions so that questionable decisions may come to the attention of the media, voters, political opponents, and law enforcements officials. These procedures should also deter questionable purchases!

The precise division of responsibility between agencies and a Purchasing Department will differ from government to government, but the lines are generally drawn based on the dollar value of a purchase and/or the type of good or service being acquired. Very expensive items or items that many agencies must buy are more likely to be acquired through central purchasing offices.

The tendency in purchasing is clearly away from informal, go-it-alone purchasing by local government departments acting independently. Instead, the trends are in the direction of centralized volume buying by professional purchasing officials acting according to standards set forth by professional associations. Centralization may involve intergovernmental agreements. In fact, a major force in local government purchasing today is buying off state contracts. In one state, for example, 80% of the purchases made under state negotiated contracts are made by local governments, not the state government. Thus, local public managers will be looking more and more to purchasing officials for assistance and service in the acquisition of the goods and services needed to administer government operations.

Cash Management

Another major aspect of the budget execution process is the cash flow of revenues and expenditures. Budgets estimate the amount of revenue to be collected and expenditures to be made

Exhibit 9-3   Investment of Short-term Cash Balances

```
        Cash management in government focuses first and foremost on the safety
of public funds, followed by liquidity considerations. In other words, cash
balances must be held in safe places and must be available for spending when
needed. When government accumulates large and continuing cash reserves, it
may be time to think about cutting taxes!

        On the other hand, it is prudent for local governments to maintain
some reserve against emergencies to avoid the unnecessary costs of short-
term borrowing if possible. Until quite recently, it was not unusual for
such reserves to be held in non-interest-paying checking accounts. Today,
many local governments actively work to consolidate fund balances in one
account and to vigorously pursue investment opportunities within the limits
set by state law as well as safety and liquidity concerns.

        Investment performance may be calculated by multiplying the amount
available for investment (cash balance) times efficiency (the percentage of
the balance invested) times the yield (rate of return on investments).
Performance may be increased by maximizing balances, consolidating funds for
investment more efficiently, or finding better investment opportunities.
Policy decisions regarding the size of cash balances and risk versus return
on investments also will affect performance.
```

over the course of the entire fiscal year. However, there is no reason to assume revenues and expenditures will flow in and out in an even balance throughout the year, or even that revenues will be collected prior to the time they are needed to meet payroll or other spending deadlines. Thus, local governments should develop cash management plans which will:

- estimate the flow of revenues and expenditures on a monthly basis (the allotment plan discussed earlier provides an estimate of expenditure flows)

- speed the collection of revenues by adjusting due dates or setting incentives for early payment or more severe penalties for late payment

- slow the disbursement of expenditures through the use of allotments and by delaying bill payments until final due dates

- minimize the costs of short-term borrowing if revenues cannot be collected prior to the time expenditures must be made. This can be accomplished by advance planning to borrow the minimum amount needed for the shortest time necessary at the most favorable rates.

- maximize short-term investment income when revenues will be received in advance of expenditure deadlines. This can be achieved by planning to invest the maximum amount possible for the longest period at the most favorable rates (see Exhibit 9-3)

Although cash management is not a direct responsibility of public managers outside of finance specialists, careful attention to cash flow enables the smooth functioning of government operations and maximizes the amount of public resources available for program operations. Therefore, it is useful for managers to have a general grasp of this important finance function which helps support their daily work.

Exhibit 9-4 Budgetary Accounting Documents and Process

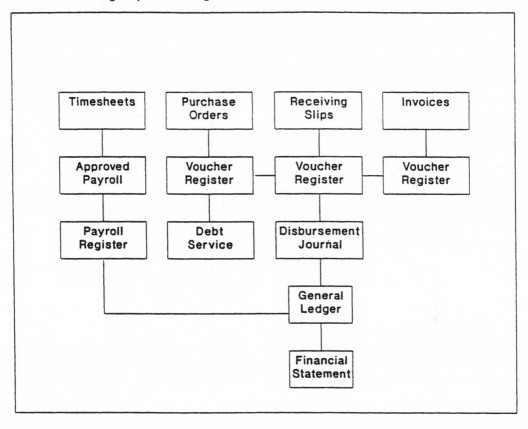

Accounting and Auditing

The various processes for spending the budget are dominated by the requirements of accounting and auditing. Although public managers often view these processes as cumbersome and time-consuming, they are the essential elements in managing the current budget and planning future budgets. Such processes also provide the control procedures and data necessary for public accountability in a democratic society:

> A fundamental tenet of a democratic society holds that governments and agencies entrusted with public resources and the authority for applying them have a responsibility to render a full accounting of their activities.[3]

Accounting provides the tools and techniques necessary for public managers to assemble, analyze, and report financial information so that it may be used for planning, decision making and control. The purpose of accounting is to provide financial information which is accurate, complete, timely, and in a form understandable to users:

> An accounting system consists of an integrated structure of source documents, journals, ledgers, and procedures used to determine the financial position of an economic

enterprise. It involves the composite activity of recording, summarizing, analyzing, and interpreting the financial transactions of any economic enterprise. It is the means by which to accomplish the goal of complete and accurate financial information that is of use to decision makers and the general public.[4]

The four parts to this structure are:

- **Source documents and forms** include such items as invoices, receipts, time cards, and purchase orders which record the details of every financial transaction including proper authorization for the action.

- **Journals** provide summary lists of all the transactions of a certain type in a chronological order, for example a payroll journal would record all payments to employees.

- **Ledgers** are based upon the summary totals in journals and show the balance in any revenue, expenditure, or other account at any time. General and subsidiary ledgers are usually used to provide different levels of detail.

- **Procedures and Controls** include the forms and instructions for classifying, recording, and reporting financial transactions in source documents, journals, and ledgers.

Exhibit 9-4[5] shows how these four parts interact in a simple accounting system.

In government, the focus of accounting is on cash flows and accountability to the entire public rather than on profit and loss as is the case in the private sector. Evolving from this basic difference are the general principles of governmental accounting (GAAP) which include the following critical concepts:

- The system should reflect whether the government has complied with all applicable legal provisions, and should fully disclose its financial condition and results of operations.

- An annual budget should be adopted and executed with unspent appropriations lapsing at the end of the fiscal year.

- Fund accounting should be used to insure legal compliance with restrictions on the use of revenues and to enhance sound financial administration of diverse governmental operations.

- Fixed assets accounts should be maintained separately from current assets. Fixed assets are not depreciated in general records except in the case of enterprise funds.

- Long-term general obligation bonds should be recorded in a separate group of accounts as obligations of the entire governmental unit. Revenue bonds are obligations of specific funds and should be recorded as such.

- Bases of accounting are methods for matching revenues and expenditures over a specified time period. On a **cash basis**, revenues are recorded when cash is received and expenditures are recorded when cash payments are actually completed. On a **full accrual basis**, revenues are recorded when earned and expenses are recorded when liability is incurred. Finally, the **modified accrual basis** records expenditures when

PRACTICAL GOVERNMENT BUDGETING

Exhibit 9-5   Auditing Terms and Concepts

o   **Audit:** an examination of systems, procedures, programs, and financial data. The end product of an audit is a report issued by an independent auditor describing how well a local government's financial statements describe its financial condition and the results of its operations.

o   **Independent Auditor:** a person or firm hired on a contractual basis who is not otherwise affiliated with the organization being audited.

o   **Compliance Audit:** determines if a local government has acted according to the applicable federal, state, and local laws, regulations, policies, and procedures.

o   **Management Audit:** determines if a local government is performing in the most economical and efficient manner, identifies possible causes for problems, and recommends methods of improvement.

o   **Program Audit:** determines whether the intended results of a local government activity are being achieved.

---

liability is incurred but does not record most revenues until cash is received. Exceptions may be made for revenues clearly measurable and available such as property taxes (particularly if the estimated revenue from this source has been reduced to account for some late or uncollectible taxes). Capital Project and Enterprise funds should be maintained on a full accrual basis, while the General Fund and other Revenue Funds should be on the more conservative modified accrual basis. Cash basis accounting, though still widely used, is not desirable since it is easier to manipulate and gives a less than complete picture of financial condition at any given point in time.

• Common language should be used throughout the budget, accounting records, and financial reports. Revenues should be classified by fund and by source, while expenditures should be recorded by fund, program, activity, and object.

• Financial reports should be issued regularly and an annual report covering all funds and operations should be prepared and published.

Audits are the device for pulling together acounting data in reports designed for particular uses and users. As noted in Exhibit 9-5, there are three possible types of audits. These audits range from the basic check for legal compliance and conformance to GAAP standards up to sophisticated management efficiency audits and program evaluation reviews.

The final part of the yearly budget cycle is the annual external audit of all government financial matters. Such regular public accounting to the citizens is, of course, the essence of the accountability demanded and appropriate in a democratic society. In addition, the annual independent audit is normally required by state law and is demanded of any jurisdiction which accepts intergovernmental aid or hopes to market bonds to fund capital projects. Although the typical public manager has little direct involvement in this auditing process, all managers share responsibility for following proper spending procedures and complying with all record-keeping requirements. In the final analysis, accounting and auditing can only be effective when original source documents are properly prepared.

EXERCISE: BUDGET EXECUTION

1. As an analyst in the central budget office, you are preparing for a mid-year budget review meeting on Patrol Services with the Chief of Police. The City Council-approved budget for the police appropriated $1.29 million for patrol, and the budget office reserved 5% for contingencies and allotted the remaining $1.225 million evenly on a monthly basis. The following data is available on the first half of the fiscal year:

Exhibit 9-6   Mid-Year Review Budget Report

Police Patrol	FY Budget	Expended	Encumbered
Personal Services:			
Salaries/Wages	$900,000	$500,000	0
Fringe Benefits	$100,000	$ 60,000	0
Operating Expenses:			
Contractual	$100,000	$ 40,000	$12,000
Supplies	$ 75,000	$ 50,000	$10,000
Capital Outlay:			
Equipment	$ 50,000	$ 10,000	$30,000
TOTALS	**$1,225,000**	**$660,000**	**$52,000**

Personal services, operating expenses, and equipment dollars cannot be shifted out of their categories without budget office approval. Expenditures in excess of the budget would require a supplemental appropriation by the council.

Considering these facts, what further research would you do before meeting with the Chief? What do you expect to ask the Chief? How do you expect her to respond? What recommendations do you anticipate making to the Budget Director regarding the budget for patrol services for the rest of the year?

2. Beach City, Maine has calculated the average number of prisoners incarcerated in the city jail over the past five years. Assuming that the city fiscal year begins April 1, please prepare quarterly allotments for the $487,800 appropriated for feeding prisoners for the upcoming fiscal year.

MONTH	PRISONERS	MONTH	PRISONERS	MONTH	PRISONERS
Jan	45	May	55	Sept	95
Feb	40	Jun	104	Oct	55
Mar	50	Jul	131	Nov	40
Apr	50	Aug	103	Dec	45

Example: On the average, there are 45 prisoners to be fed each day in the month of January.

3. A city's cash management plan anticipated an average amount available for investment of $5 million with an efficiency rate of 95% at an average yield of 10%. At the end of the fiscal year, data reveals an average amount available of $4.5 million, an efficiency rate of 97.5% and an average yield of 10.5%. How well did the city do on its investments compared to plan? What caused the variance from the plan? Did the individual in charge of cash management do a good job?

```
NOTES
```

1. *An Operating Budget Handbook for Small Cities and Governmental Units* (Chicago, Illinois: Municipal Finance Officers Association, 1978), pp. 82-83.

2. Penelope Lemov, "Evolution in Purchasing," *Governing,* Vol. I, No. 11 (August 1988), pp. 43-44.

3. Comptroller General of the U.S., *Standards of Audit of Government Organizations, Programs, Activities and Functions* (Washington D.C.: U. S. General Accounting Office, 1974), pp. 1-2.

4. Robert A. Reny, "Municipal Accounting," in Jack Rabin *et al,* editors, *Budget Management* (Athens, Georgia: Carl Vinson Institute of Government, 1983), p. 128.

5. *Costing and Pricing Municipal Services* (Boston, Massachusetts: Commonwealth of Massachusetts Executive Office of Communities and Development, August, 1982), p. 20.

Chapter 10

MULTI-YEAR BUDGETS

The Case For a Multi-Year Budget Perspective

HOW THIS CHAPTER WILL BE USEFUL

Local governments are ongoing organizations and the services they provide generally continue for many years. Thus, today's decisions about raising revenues and funding programs usually affect the locality's budget for years to come. In any particular year, the total impact of the taxing and spending choices of previous years is far more important in shaping the final budget document than any new decisions made in the annual budget preparation process.

Nonetheless, the traditional local government outlook has been that "Short-term planning is the next budget; long-term planning is the next election."[1] Efforts to estimate revenues and expenditures for several years into the future have been dismissed by observations such as "we don't have the time," "nobody cares anyway," and "it can't be done with enough accuracy to make it worthwhile."

This perspective has been changing rapidly in the past decade or so. Even middle-sized and small cities and counties have begun to develop, implement, and report what are usually called "Five Year Financial Forecasts." There are a number of reasons for this change in attitude:

- In political terms, both big deficits and big surpluses are often viewed in negative terms:

  ...the administration that permits the state to slide into a deficit position is ineffective, wild-spending, and mismanaged. The administration that produces a surplus has overtaxed the people, been stingy with social programs, and is probably planning an election-year tax cut.[2]

- When considered on a one-year basis, the budget often seems out of control. Personnel costs, building maintenance and operations, mandated programs, and even discretionary activities can be legally or politically impossible to change in any given year.

- Affordable computer hardware and software has considerably eased the burden of establishing and especially updating financial forecasts.

Therefore, local governments have taken to multi-year projections as a feasible method of gaining more control over their budgets, particularly in order to anticipate and thus avoid major deficits or surpluses.

For line and staff local public administrators, the use of multi-year budget projections has two important implications:

- First, agency and program planning and operations can take place in a more informed setting, since agency officials can better anticipate the local government's future financial position.

- Second, the same techniques and processes used to develop macro-level projections for the whole city or county can also be used to estimate the future expenditure requirements of micro-level agency or program activities.

OBJECTIVES

In sum, the use of five-year projections of income and spending is spreading rapidly to local governments. It is going to be increasingly important for public managers to:

1. Understand the development, uses, and limitations of these projections.

2. Apply government-wide estimates to their particular agency management tasks.

3. Utilize projection techniques to plan and justify agency spending requests on a multi-year basis.

This chapter should introduce the reader to the knowledge, skills, and abilities needed to master these three objectives.

MULTI-YEAR
FORECASTING AND PLANNING

The Benefits of Looking Ahead

Multi-year budget projecting is

a financial management / financial planning tool which provides management at all levels with information on the long-term fiscal implications of current policies, programs, and economic and planning assumptions.[3]

Such forecasted information is neither a prediction about the future nor a statement of policy intentions. Instead, forecasts are estimates of the future impact of current revenue and expenditure policies based upon specific assumptions about future conditions such as inflation

or population growth. Generally, local government financial forecasts are "rolling" five-year projections, meaning that the figures are updated and revised annually.

There are a number of possible benefits derived from establishing and using a multi-year forecasting process:

- Forecasts provide advance warning of potential budget imbalances before a crisis stage is reached and drastic, quick-fix measures are the only resort.

- Forecasts improve the quality of all revenue and spending policy decisions of chief executives and legislative bodies by supplying additional information about financial implications beyond the immediate fiscal year.

- Forecasts assist agency managers, rank-and-file public employees, citizens, interest groups, and the local media in understanding the jurisdiction's financial condition and its implications for specific policy decisions. Thus, forecasts may help build support for painful decisions regarding tax increases or spending reductions.

Financial Forecasts and Gap Analysis

One of the principal uses and motivating forces behind financial forecasts is to examine the prospects for revenue collections and program expenditures five years into the future in order to identify "gaps." These "gaps" represent unbalanced budgets which are forecast in one or more of the coming fiscal years unless spending can be cut or revenues increased.

On a multi-year basis, revenue sources are projected individually in much the same manner as discussed in Chapter 6. However, several additional assumptions are necessary, which typically include:

- tax rates and charges for licenses, fees, and permits will remain constant over the forecast period

- no new taxes or other revenue sources will be developed

- revenue growth can be projected with sufficient accuracy for planning purposes several years into the future.

These first two assumptions can be adjusted, of course, to accommodate changes in sources or rates of revenue which have already been scheduled for future implementation. Generally, though, forecasts project the future outcomes of current local government budgetary policies and decisions, and do not attempt to anticipate what local decision makers will do in the future.

Five-year revenue projections can be based upon statistical relationships to economic factors such as the consumer price index or demographic projections, historical revenue growth trends, and expert judgement.

For example, some revenue sources may be closely tied to particular economic variables which economists expend enormous efforts to try to predict. Thus, local government revenues from interest earnings can be projected based upon anticipated interest rates while sales tax receipts can be calculated from economists' predictions of retail sales and other economic activity subject to the sales tax. Other revenue sources may be estimated with confidence based upon clear and continuing historical patterns. Thus, if parking fines have increased about 5% annually for the last five years and there are no reasons to expect any changes in the parking situation in the foreseeable future, one can

Exhibit 10-1   Using Trends to Forecast Revenues

    A simple way to estimate future income from revenue sources is to project future year collections on the basis of historical trends. This method assumes that past trends will continue during the forecast period. For example, assume a city has received the following income over the past six years from rental of its civic center to community groups:

        FY 1982 - $36,894   FY 1985 - $43,422
        FY 1983 - 39,552   FY 1986 - 43,568
        FY 1984 - 41,937   FY 1987 - 45,711

    Because the revenue source is not large and the the basic assumption that we can use the past five years to estimate the next five years is less than certain, a simple step-by-step approach is most reasonable:

o   Determine the absolute change in collections each year (From 1982 to 1983, revenues increased by $39,552 minus $36,894 equals $2658).

o   Determine the percentage change each year (From 1982 to 1983, divide $2658 by $36,894 to equal 7.2%).

o   Add the percentage changes and divide by the number of changes (Here, there are five changes to be determined, totaled and divided by 5 to get average percent change).

o   Multiply the average percent change (assume it works out to exactly 5%) times each of the first five fiscal years in the example and compare results to the actual collections. (A 5% increase from 1982 collections of $36,894 equals $38,738. The actual 1983 collections of $39,552 can then be divided by the "projected" 1983 collections of $38,738 and multiplied by 100 which equals 102%. This means actual collections were just a bit more than projected revenues. As long as this "percentage of projection" is fairly close to 100%, one can conclude that a trend is present. Thus, this step is a "check" on whether the trend method is appropriate.

o   Finally, the average percent change is multiplied by the most recent year's collections to project the following year and so on. (In this example, a 5% increase in our 1987 revenues equals the 1988 projection, a 5% increase in the 1988 projection equals 1989's estimate, and so on).

estimate annual 5% increases in this revenue source. Finally, some revenue forecasts must rely entirely on expert judgement. A good example is intergovernmental aid. Essentially, local officials must assess the national or state political and fiscal climate in order to guess the future intentions of higher-level policy makers regarding contraction, continuation, or expansion of aid programs.

Because of the uncertainty surrounding any and all of these methods, local government financial forecasts must always be considered rough guesses rather than precise measures. Generally, local governments use historical trend analysis (see Exhibit 10-1) or simple statistical relationships (see Exhibit 10-2). Professional judgement is utilized when the future is deemed unlikely to follow past patterns, data is nonexistent or of uncertain quality, or if analysis does not reveal clear trends or relationships. Many jurisdictions utilize more than one set of economic assumptions to produce, for example, best-case and worst-case revenue projections.

Future expenditures are estimated by methods explained in Chapter 2 and 3 along with several other assumptions such as:

Exhibit 10-2   Example of Statistical Projection

```
        Statistical projection methods rely on the presumed relationship of
    the revenue source to some other quantity whose future value can be better
    estimated.

        For example, the best way to estimate the future value of many revenue
    sources is to rely on their relationship to changes in population. The
    advantages are several: population projections are the subject of much
    analysis, they are easily available, and they often have a logical
    relationship to many revenues and expenditures. Over the years, these
    relationships may be statistically validated but, in the real world, local
    government officials usually must rely on their judgement to decide if these
    relationships hold true for their particular jurisdiction.

o   Once the data is gathered and the relationship is determined, the
    actual calculations are quite simple. For example, let's assume that
    there is a perfect correlation between population change and fee
    collections for hunting and fishing licenses. Revenues from these fees
    in FfY 1989 were $12,373. Population projections for the next few years
    are:

            FY 1990   +2.9%      FY 1993   +3.5%
            FY 1991   +3.0%      FY 1994   +2.4%
            FY 1992   +2.8%      FY 1995   +2.1%

o   Since we believe that the best available method of estimating this
    source is to assume it varies exactly as does population, simply
    multiply the change in population times the previous year's actual or
    estimated collections to obtain the next year's projection.

o   From this example, collections for FY 1990 would be estimated at 1.029
    (100% for the previous year's collections and 2.9% for the anticipated
    increase) times FY 1989 fees of $12,373, which equals $12,732. This new
    figure would be multiplied by 1.03 for FY 1991 etc.
```

- no changes in government personnel or service levels of existing programs will occur

- no new services or programs will be provided

- expenditure growth can be forecast based upon anticipated changes in the costs of personnel, operating expenses, and capital outlay items. As with revenues, a combination of statistical analysis, projection of past trends, and informed judgement is usually used to determine the rates of growth in spending. The choice of specific techniques for forecasting expenditures (or revenues) will vary based upon staff and other resources, available data, and the importance of the item being projected. A major expenditure item such as salaries will be scrutinized with more care than a minor item.

Once revenue and expenditure projections are produced for the five succeeding years, they are usually presented in a "Gap Analysis" format such as the example shown in Exhibit 10-3.[4] This example reveals a possible future of annual budget deficits growing from $5.849 million in 1979-1980 to $17.818 million in 1983-1984 if current revenue and expenditure policies remain unchanged. The figures in the boxes indicate the **permanent increases in revenues or permanent decreases in expenditures** needed to balance the budget. If such steps are taken annually, then the size of the tax increase or spending cutback which will be needed in 1983-1984, for example, drops from $17.818 million to only $2.867 million.

Exhibit 10-3   An Example of Gap Analysis

Fiscal	1989-90	1990-91	1991-92	1992-93	1993-94	5 Year Effect of Reducing Budget
1989-90	$ 5,849	6,321	6,645	7,419	8,055	$34,489
1990-91		1,920	2,078	2,252	2,444	8,694
1991-92			1,674	1,813	1,967	5,454
1992-93				2,289	2,485	4,774
1993-94					2,867	2,867
Additional Resources Needed to Provide 1988-89 Level of Services	5,849	8,241	10,597	13,773	17,818	56,278

* Numbers underlined equal the combination of additional permanent new revenues and permanent new expenditure reductions needed to balance each fiscal year's budget (in 000/s of dollars). For example, in 1989-90, $5,849,000 in permanent cuts or new taxes are needed to balance the budget. If this is done, in 1990-91, $1,920,000 will be needed. If, on the other hand, one time cuts or revenues are used to balance the 1989-90 budget, there will be a continuing shortfall of $6,321,000 ($5,849,000 times anticipated inflation) as well as the new $1,920,000 imbalance. Thus the total needed to balance the 1990-91 budget would be $8,241,000.

Exhibit 10-3 assumes annual inflation rates of slightly over 8%. Thus, if decision-makers do not enact permanent tax and fee hikes for FY 1989-80 or make permanent cuts in the budget, the $5.8 million shortfall will increase by 8% to a $6.3 million deficit in 1980-81. On top of that, the projections of spending and revenue trends indicate that there will be an additional $1.9 million imbalance in FY1980-81, for a total deficit of $8.2 million.

Gap analysis thus represents the purposes of financial forecasts very well. It is not intended to predict a series of future deficits; after all local governments are legally required to balance their budgets. It is certainly not designed to recommend a five-year succession of increasingly serious shortfalls in the budget. Rather, **the goal of gap analysis is to enable decision makers to assess the current situation in a broader context and to make today's decisions in light of the needs of both the immediate situation and the future.**

In the particular case presented in Exhibit 10-3, for instance, local government officials preparing the budget for FY 1989-80 are faced with increasing revenues by $5.8 million or reducing services by a like amount. In the absence of a five-year forecast, officials might be tempted to sell land, institute a hiring freeze, enact a one-year tax increase, postpone maintenance of capital facilities, or take other temporary, one-time solutions to address the immediate $5.8 million imbalance in the budget. Even if these measures were successful in addressing that year's financial emergency, by the next year officials would be facing an even bigger $8.2 million deficit crisis! The Five-Year Gap Analysis thus offers the insight necessary to show decision makers that in this situation, a more permanent solution to the 1979-1980 deficit is in order.

Impact Analysis of Budgetary Decisions

The other major type of multi-year budget projection technique is the estimation of the long-term financial impact of particular policy decisions. This kind of analysis is routinely done with major capital projects, particularly those which are to be financed with revenue bonds. Anticipated revenues from the completed project must be adequate to pay off the bonds issued to finance construction of the facility!

However, impact analysis can also be important whenever new policy goals are adopted, new programs are instituted, or new performance standards are established. Methods of projections are basically identical to those used in gap analysis. Agency officials in most local governments will be called upon to produce such analyses in the next few years if they are not already doing so. Examples might include estimating the impact on the budget for the next five years if:

- A new policy of waiving recreation fees for senior citizens is adopted.

- A new program to provide after-school care for community children is instituted.

- A new performance standard of responding to all nonemergency police calls within 15 minutes is established.

A detailed approach to estimating the net impact on an agency budget of various possible additional service commitments is shown in Exhibit 10-4. Note that the "department" budget can grow as the result of:

- The higher cost of providing the same services as the previous year at the coming year's higher prices (inflators).

- The addition of new activities and responsibilites (program change).

- A higher or improved level of quality in providing the same services as the previous year (change in service level).

- Providing the same services at the same level as the previous year to a larger number of service recipients (change in work base).

- Staffing and operating a new building or other capital facility (new facility operating costs).

Thus, as any of these actions is contemplated, it is appropriate to do an impact analysis to project the financial implications of such decisions for future year budgets.

Multi-Year Planning For Cyclical Expenditures

Although local government budgets are usually prepared on an annual basis, not all local expenditures fall neatly into annual cycles. Equipment is the major example of this phenomenon. For

Exhibit 10-4   A Model for Expenditure Forecasting

> A comprehensive attempt to estimate spending for a governmental unit such as a bureau or department can be a complex undertaking. There are numerous factors which can cause increases or decreases in the unit's projected expenditures. A simple formula to determine the overall impact of various possible changes is:
>
> o   Prior year (or estimated current year) expenditures, times
>
> o   The rate of inflation and/or changes in salaries and wages, plus/minus
>
> o   Costs of new programs added or old programs eliminated, plus/minus
>
> o   Costs of increasing/decreasing the level or quality of services, plus/minus
>
> o   Costs of extending/reducing the scope of services to new areas or additional clients, plus/minus
>
> o   Costs of operating new/closed facilities, plus/minus
>
> o   Productivity gains/losses
>
> In sum, consideration of all these factors should give the best possible estimate of future levels of spending by a particular budget unit by incorporating the impact of all significant changes in operations.

instance, motor vehicles represent costly capital outlay purchases which are presumed to have a useful life longer than one year. In order to avoid irregular strains on budgets in years when vehicles must be replaced, a multi-year budget perspective is necessary to plan a method of spreading costs of acquisitions evenly across the fiscal years.

Several methods of accomplishing this goal are used by local governments:[5]

- Large equipment items may be purchased through a capital equipment pool of funds financed by a bond issue, thus equalizing costs over the period of years the equipment will be used.

- A purchasing schedule could be established along with an annual budget line item for an equipment reserve fund adequate to meet replacement costs for equipment as its useful life expires.

- A formal plan could be designed so that large cyclical purchases are staggered over the years with roughly equal amounts expended on capital outlay each year.

- Interagency internal service funds may be used to purchase and maintain certain types of equipment such as autombiles for the entire local government. This broader base allows a smoother purchase schedule and separates agency operating budgets from confusing, irregular peaks and valleys due to cyclical capital outlay patterns. Operating agencies are then billed for actual use of equipment, which probably results in a much more regular and predictable expenditure picture.

Any of these solutions will alleviate the necessity for agencies to make occasional major demands for extra funds for expensive equipment. This can be especially helpful since such demands are often delayed until the items are absolutely necessary, regardless of the fiscal or political outlook of the particular budget season. For the local government as a whole, smoothing out the funding of capital outlay equipment makes budget planning an easier and more manageable process.

The Politics of Multi-Year Forecasts

As is the case with all public management tools, the use of financial forecasts has political implications as well as with the ability to improve the technical quality of budget decision making.

Obviously, clearly communicated financial projections may have the effect of encouraging or discouraging new expenditure proposals. Therefore, advocates of new spending may then try to portray dismal estimates of future budget deficits as inaccurate. Since responsible local governments will act to avoid the projected budget deficits, the spending advocates later will appear to have been accurate! A particular version of this general problem occurs with the question of salaries and fringe benefits. Especially in cities and counties where employees bargain collectively for wages and benefits, the figures used for forecasting may be considered as the "minimum opening offer" by the government employer rather than an estimate based on typical wage patterns.

An even more immediate problem may occur when financial forecasts of future budgetary imbalances lead to political charges of overspending or overtaxing in election years. In such situations, public officials should be receiving praise for seeking to gather, analyze, and act on a five-year planning basis. In fact, forecasts may be used (often inaccurately and inappropriately!) as ammunition by political opponents.

Problems like these cannot be avoided completely, and therefore political considerations may at times become part of the forecasting calculations themselves in a sort of self-fulfilling prophecy. However, the more desirable solution is for the forecast to focus on the analysis of choices available to local policy makers to deal with the forecasted outcomes, rather than on the precise accuracy of the projections.

Given that forecasts are at least one step removed from the immediate budget preparation battles, there is a slightly improved chance that the politicization of projections can be held to a minimum in many jurisdictions.

Conclusion

One of the biggest problems in public budgeting and in government generally is that the incentives are very strong for many key actors to adopt a short-term outlook despite the fact that they are dealing with issues and decisions with significant long-term impacts on the communities they serve. Multi-year budget forecasts provide an important device for encouraging a longer-term perspective on the annual budget process.

☑ EXERCISE: MULTI-YEAR FORECASTS

1. Complete the trend analysis to forecast civic center rental fees presented in Exhibit 10-1. Draw a graph showing the historical data and the future projections. Are you comfortable with these projections? Why or why not?

2. Complete the statistical projection of hunting and fishing license fees described in Exhibit 10-2. Draw a graph showing the historical data and the future projections. Are you comfortable with the results? Why or why not?

3. Assume you are the Director of Parks and Recreation and you have just received a copy of your government's Five Year Forecast. The report includes the Gap Analysis displayed in this chapter as Exhibit 10-3. The total government operating budget for 1979-1980 is forecast at $98.6 million. What would your strategy be in developing your agency budget plans for 1979-1980 and subsequent years?

4. Assume that you are the Budget Director in the same situation as described in #3 above. What policy options would you present to the Mayor and City Council for addressing the issues raised by the Gap Analysis? Note that the 1979-1980 budget must be adopted two months prior to the coming municipal election.

NOTES

1. Carol W. Lewis and A. Grayson Walker III, *Casebook in Public Budgeting and Financial Management* (Englewood Cliffs, New Jersey: Prentice-Hall, 1984), p. 265.

2. Leo V. Donohue, "Confessions of a Budgeteer," in Carol W. Lewis and A. Grayson Walker III, *Casebook in Public Budgeting and Financial Management* (Englewood Cliffs, New Jersey: Prentice-Hall, 1984), p. 267.

3. *Multi-Year Revenue and Expenditure Forecasting* (Washington, D.C.: Public Technology Incorporated, 1980), p. 11.

4. *Ibid.*, p. 16.

5. *An Operating Budget Handbook for Small Cities and Governmental Units* (Chicago, Illinois: Municipal Finance Officers Associations, 1978), pp. 82-83.